Essentials of
ELECTRONIC
HEALTH RECORDS

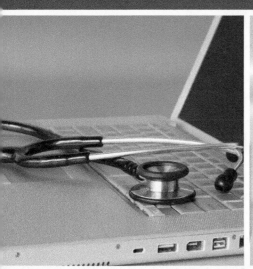
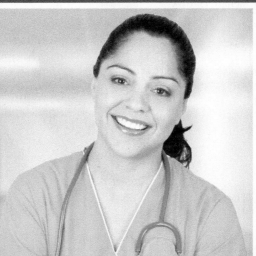
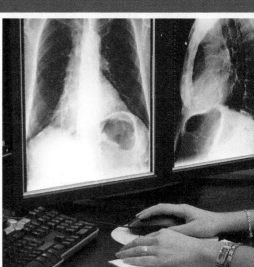

Richard Gartee

Publisher: Julie Levin Alexander
Publisher's Assistant: Regina Bruno
Editor-in-Chief: Mark Cohen
Executive Editor: Joan Gill
Associate Editor: Bronwen Glowacki
Editorial Assistant: Mary Ellen Ruitenberg
Developmental Editor: Jill Rembetski
Director of Marketing: David Gesell
Senior Marketing Manager: Katrin Beacom
Marketing Specialist: Michael Sirinides
Marketing Assistant: Crystal Gonzalez
Managing Production Editor: Patrick Walsh
Production Liaison: Julie Boddorf
Production Editor: Peggy Kellar
Senior Media Editor: Amy Peltier
Media Project Manager: Lorena Cerisano
Manufacturing Manager: Alan Fischer
Senior Art Director: Maria Guglielmo
Cover Designer: Rachael Cronin
Cover Images: iStockphoto
Composition: Aptara®, Inc.
Printing and Binding: RR Donnelley
Cover Printer: Lehigh-Phoenix Color

CPT-4® is a registered trademark of the American Medical Association
EXCEL®, Windows 2000®, Windows XP®, Windows Vista®, and Windows 7® are a registered trademarks of Microsoft Corporation
Google™ is a trademark of Google, Inc.
IMPAC is a trademark of IMPAC Medical Systems, Inc.
IQmark™ is a trademark of Midmark Diagnostics Group
LOINC® is a registered trademark of the Regenstrief Institute
Lotus 1-2-3® is a registered trademark of International Business Machines, Corp.
MEDCIN® is a registered trademark of Medicomp Systems, Inc.
The Medical Manager, Intergy, and OmniDoc™ are trademarks of Sage Software Healthcare, Inc.
NextGen® is a registered trademark of NextGen Healthcare Information Systems, Inc.
SNOMED® and SNOMED CT® are registered trademarks of the College of American Pathologists
WebMD, WebMD Health, and Medscape are trademarks of WebMD, Inc.
All other trademarks are the property of their respective owners.

Library of Congress Cataloging-in-Publication Data
Gartee, Richard.
   Essentials of electronic health records / Richard Gartee.
      p. ; cm.
   ISBN-13: 978-0-13-708525-5
   ISBN-10: 0-13-708525-7
   1. Medical records—Data processing.   I. Title.
   [DNLM: 1. Electronic Health Records—Problems and Exercises.
2. Forms and Records Control—methods—Problems and Exercises.   WX 18.2]
   R864.G372 2010
   610.285—dc22
                                    2010046540

12 11 10 9 8

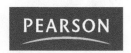

www.pearsonhighered.com

ISBN 10:   0-13-708525-7
ISBN 13: 978-0-13-708525-5

for Joan

Contents

Preface

Introduction

Almost daily the media makes us aware that healthcare needs to and *is* making a transition from paper to electronic health records (EHR). Government incentive programs have increased the rate at which electronic health records are being adopted and set a target date of 2015 for complete transition. The result is that virtually every allied health professional is going to need to understand and be able to use electronic health records.

This book answers that need by providing a short, but thorough introduction to the history, theory, and potential benefits of electronic health records. The combination of this text and the accompanying EHR software provides a complete learning system. Guided hands-on exercises using the Student Edition software provide practical experience that leads to an understanding and a level of comfort with computerized medical records that can be applied directly to the healthcare workplace. Critical thinking hands-on exercises build confidence by allowing the students to apply what they have learned.

Hands-on exercises are not aimed at teaching a particular brand of medical records software but, rather, at providing the student with practical experiences using an EHR. The software used with this book is based on Medcin®, one of the nationally accepted nomenclature standards. Because more than 15 of the top ambulatory EHR systems use the Medcin nomenclature, the skills acquired by completing the exercises are transferable to many prominent EHR systems. Even EHR systems that may use proprietary or user-defined nomenclatures still behave in a conceptually similar way to the EHR software provided with this book. These facts increase the likelihood that the student's knowledge will transfer easily to a commercial medical record system in use at a clinic.

In closing, let me offer a few words of advice:

◆ When you print a document, be certain you have your printout in hand before exiting the software. Computers "spool" print jobs, so it may seem like the application has finished printing, but your pages may not have been printed yet.

◆ Every exercise can be completed in a normal class session. When you finish an exercise, consider the amount of class time remaining before beginning the next exercise.

◆ The comprehensive exam exercise in Chapter 9 may require the full class time for the exercise. Consider the amount of class time remaining after the written exam before beginning the comprehensive exercise.

The purpose of this book is to enable schools to introduce electronic health records in a curriculum where the allotted time does not permit a longer full-length EHR course. This limitation means, of course, that there is substantially more that you can learn about electronic health records.

- If you enjoy what you learn here, ask your school if the full EHR course is offered.

- You may also wish to purchase the full-length book *Electronic Health Records: Understanding and Using Computerized Medical Records,* 2nd edition (ISBN: 0132499762). The full-length book uses the same software as this text and has more than 75 exercises.

The Development and Organization of the Text

This book is organized to provide learners with a comprehensive understanding. Each chapter builds on the knowledge acquired in previous chapters. Chapters 2 through 9 reinforce the material with practical experiences using electronic health record software.

Chapter 1: Electronic Health Records—An Overview provides a foundation for student learning, introducing the fundamental requirements and reasons for electronic health records. The chapter begins with a definition of electronic health records and then discusses why they are important and the forces in our society driving their adoption. Workflow scenarios compare the flow of information when using paper versus electronic charts. Critical thinking exercises challenge the learner to analyze workflow.

Chapter 2: Functional EHR Systems describes the various forms of storing EHR data and the value of using standardized codes for that data. The chapter covers the prominent nomenclature standards and their history, purpose, and relationship to each other. Hands-on exercises allow the students to explore a common component of most EHR systems, the document imaging system. Additional Chapter 2 topics include the potential uses of EHR data for patient health management, decision support, and the electronic interchange of data between systems.

Chapter 3: Learning Medical Record Software introduces the Medcin Student Edition software, which will be used for the remainder of the book. In a series of brief hands-on exercises, the student becomes familiar with EHR concepts, learns to navigate the software, and creates an actual encounter note.

Chapter 4: Increased Familiarity with the Software reinforces the student's computer skills with additional hands-on exercises. Students also learn how to save their work as printed encounters or output encounter notes to PDF or XPS files.

Chapter 5: Learning to Use Search and Prompt continues to build on the previous chapters and teaches students how to quickly locate medical findings. Additionally, students are introduced to computerized order entry and electronic orders. Hands-on exercises are used for each feature.

Chapter 6: Learning to Use Lists teaches students a method of documenting routine encounters that is used in almost all EHR systems to speed data entry. Chapter 6 also introduces the student to electronic prescriptions, which are now required in all certified EHR systems.

Chapter 7: Entering EHR Data Using Forms covers another method of data entry that is found in most commercial EHR systems, forms. The chapter compares the two methods, Lists and Forms, and the student learns through hands-on exercises using an electronic standard initial visit intake form, and then in a subsequent hands-on exercise learns to combine both the List and Form methods of data entry.

One very practical fact of healthcare is that providers need to be paid for their work. The vast majority of those payments are realized by filing insurance claims that require the use of standardized codes.

Chapter 8: EHR Coding and Reimbursement discusses the ICD-9-CM diagnoses, CPT-4, and HCPCS codes sets. Hands-on exercises with EHR software allow the student to explore the relationship of the encounter note to the evaluation and management billing codes. Guided exercises simplify complicated billing rules through practical experience.

Chapter 9: Comprehensive Evaluation provides learners with a comprehensive measure of their understanding by combining a written examination with an extensive hands-on exercise using EHR software.

Learning Made Easy

A Unique Approach to Learning the Essentials of Electronic Health Records

This textbook-software package introduces learners to the electronic health record (EHR) through practical applications and guided exercises. The textbook and Medcin Student Edition software combination provides a complete learning system. Chapters integrate the history, theory, and benefits of EHR with the opportunity to experience the EHR environment firsthand by completing guided exercises and critical thinking exercises using the Student Edition software. Each chapter builds on the knowledge acquired in previous chapters.

Applying Theory to Practice

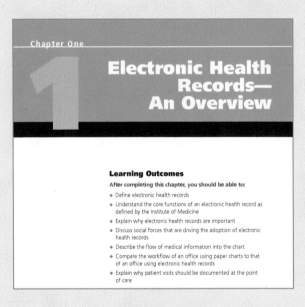

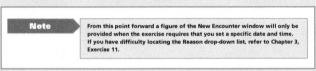

Note From this point forward a figure of the New Encounter window will only be provided when the exercise requires that you set a specific date and time. If you have difficulty locating the Reason drop-down list, refer to Chapter 3, Exercise 11.

NOTES Note boxes found within the chapters explain key terms that are used within the text and provide additional information about the software.

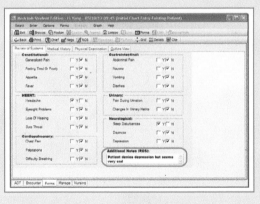

LEARNING OUTCOMES Each chapter begins with a list of learning outcomes that highlight the key concepts contained in that chapter.

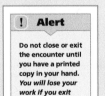

! Alert

Do not close or exit the encounter until you have a printed copy in your hand. You will lose your work if you exit before printing.

ALERTS Alert boxes found within the chapters caution or remind learners about information related to using the software.

Chapter Four Summary

In this chapter you have performed exercises intended to increase your familiarity with the Student Edition software and thereby increase your speed of data entry. You have also learned how to print out encounter notes or export them as files. You can print the encounter note at any time and as often as you like while practicing your exercises. However, remember not to quit or exit the program until you are sure the encounter note has printed. Once you exit, you will lose your work.

As you continue through the course you can refer to the Exercise 27 in this chapter if you need to remember how to print or export a file. You can also repeat any of the exercises in this chapter to increase your skills using the software. You should not proceed with the remainder of the text until you can perform the exercises in this chapter with ease.

CHAPTER SUMMARY Summaries at the end of each chapter synthesize key points for students and include a reference table of exercises that cover specific EHR skills.

Practice Opportunities

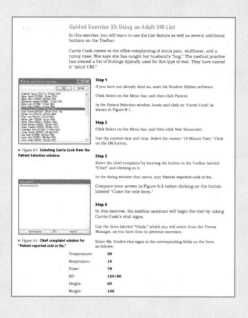

Guided Exercise 33: Using an Adult URI List

In this exercise, you will learn to use the List feature as well as several additional buttons on the Toolbar.

Carrie Cook comes to the office complaining of sinus pain, stuffiness, and a runny nose. She says she has caught her husband's "bug." The medical practice has created a list of findings typically used for this type of visit. They have named it "Adult URI."

Step 1
If you have not already done so, start the Student Edition software.
Click Select on the Menu bar, and then click Patient.
In the Patient Selection window, locate and click on "Carrie Cook" as shown in Figure 6-1.

► Figure 6-1 **Selecting Carrie Cook from the Patient Selection window.**

Step 2
Click Select on the Menu bar, and then click New Encounter.
Use the current date and time. Select the reason "10 Minute Visit." Click on the OK button.

Step 3
Enter the chief complaint by locating the button in the Toolbar labeled "Chief" and clicking on it.
In the dialog window that opens, type Patient reported cold or flu.
Compare your screen to Figure 6-2 before clicking on the button labeled "Close the note form."

Step 4
In this exercise, the medical assistant will begin the visit by taking Carrie Cook's vital signs.
Use the form labeled "Vitals," which you will select from the Forms Manager, as you have done in previous exercises.

► Figure 6-2 **Chief complaint window for "Patient reported cold or flu."**

Enter Ms. Cook's vital signs in the corresponding fields on the form as follows:

Temperature:	99
Respiration:	16
Pulse:	78
BP:	120/80
Height:	60
Weight:	100

◄ **GUIDED EXERCISES** Guided exercises that use a step-by-step approach allow the student to learn by doing. The companion Medcin Student Edition software provides a computer experience similar to that of an actual medical facility.

Critical Thinking Exercise 29: A Patient with Sinusitis

This exercise will help you evaluate how well you can use the Student Edition software to create an encounter note. The exercise provides step-by-step instructions, but does not provide screen figures for reference. The exercises in Chapter 3 covered each feature used in this exercise. If you have difficulty at any step during this exercise, refer to the Chapter 3 Summary where a table lists each feature and the corresponding exercise for that feature.

Patient John Lewis has been experiencing stuffy sinus pain. The medical office has scheduled a brief office visit for him to see the nurse practitioner. Using what you have learned so far, document Mr. Lewis's brief exam.

Step 1
If you have not already done so, start the Student Edition software.
Click Select on the Menu bar, and then click Patient.
In the Patient Selection window, locate and click on "John Lewis."

Step 2
Click Select on the Menu bar, and then click New Encounter.
Select the reason "10 minute visit" from the drop-down list.
Make sure you have selected the reason correctly. You may use the current date for this exercise.

Step 3
Enter the chief complaint by locating the button in the Toolbar labeled "Chief" and clicking on it.
In the dialog window that opens, type Stuffy sinus.
Click on the button labeled "Close the note form."

Step 4
The patient reports a sinus pain, stuffy nose, and nasal discharge. Enter the patient's symptoms using the list of findings on the Sx tab:

◄ **CRITICAL THINKING EXERCISES** Hands-on critical thinking exercises challenge learners to extend what they have learned through their completion of the guided exercises by applying their knowledge in a new way.

► **TESTING YOUR KNOWLEDGE** Open-ended study questions at the end of each chapter allow learners to test their knowledge and think critically.

Testing Your Knowledge of Chapter 6

You may run the Medcin Student Edition software and use your mouse on the screen to answer the following questions:

1. How do you select a list?
2. Name one of the advantages of using a list.
3. What Entry Details field is used with a finding to indicate the patient's fever was "mild"?

Write the meaning of each of the following medical abbreviations as they were used in this chapter.

4. ROS
5. HPI _____

6. HEENT _____
7. URI _____
8. Sig _____
9. What is the effect of selecting Sx findings with the ROS button on?
10. What is the effect of selecting Sx findings with the ROS button off?
11. The Auto Negative (Nega) button functions on what two tabs?
12. Which button on the Toolbar invokes the prescription writer?
13. Which section of the SOAP note is a prescription written into?
14. Which section of the encounter note is allergy information written into?
15. You should have produced two narrative documents of patient encounters, which you printed. If you have not already done so, hand these in to your instructor with this test. The printed encounter notes will count as a portion of your grade.

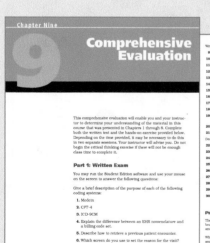

Chapter Nine

9 Comprehensive Evaluation

This comprehensive evaluation will enable you and your instructor to determine your understanding of the material in this course that was presented in Chapters 1 through 8. Complete both the written test and the hands-on exercise provided below. Depending on the time provided, it may be necessary to do this in two separate sessions. Your instructor will advise you. Do not begin the critical thinking exercise if there will not be enough class time to complete it.

Part 1: Written Exam

You may run the Student Edition software and use your mouse on the screen to answer the following questions:

Give a brief description of the purpose of each of the following coding systems:

1. Medcin
2. CPT-4
3. ICD-9CM
4. Explain the difference between an EHR nomenclature and a billing code set.
5. Describe how to retrieve a previous patient encounter.
6. Which screen do you use to set the reason for the visit?
7. How do you load a list?
8. How do you enter vital signs?

Write the meaning of each of the following medical abbreviations:

9. ROS _____
10. Hx _____
11. HEENT _____
12. Dx _____
13. PFSH _____
14. URI _____
15. E&M _____
16. Describe how to record a test that was performed.
17. How many levels are there for a category of E&M codes?
18. Name the key components of an E&M code.
19. What Entry Details field is used with a finding to indicate a "possible" diagnosis?
20. What determines the E&M level of risk?
21. Where are "bullets" as used in E&M calculations?

Describe the purpose of the following buttons on the Medcin Toolbar:

22. Prompt _____
23. Order _____
24. Listsize _____
25. Rx _____
26. Search _____
27. Nega _____
28. ROS _____
29. E&M _____
30. Explain the difference between calculating the E&M level of a general multi-system examination and a single-organ examination.

Part 2: Critical Thinking Exercise

The following exercise will use features of the software with which you have become familiar. Complete each step in sequential order using the instructions and other information provided.

When you have finished the complete exercise, print out the encounter note and hand it to your instructor. Do not begin the hands-on exercise if there will not be enough class time to complete it.

Critical Thinking Exercise 42: Examination of a Patient with Asthma

George Blackstone is a 30-year-old established patient with possible mild asthma who comes to the office complaining of awakening in the night short of breath. George does not smoke, but he is exposed to second-hand smoke and has pets in the house.

In this exercise, you use the skills you have acquired to document this exam.

Step 1
If you have not already done so, start the Student Edition software.
Click Select on the Menu bar, and then click Patient.
In the Patient Selection window, locate and click on "George Blackstone."

Step 2
Click Select on the Menu bar, and then click New Encounter.
Select the date "May 14, 2012," the time "9:15 AM," and the reason "10 Minute Visit."
Make certain that you set the date and reason correctly. Compare your screen to the date, time, and reason given above before clicking on the OK button.

Step 3
Enter the chief complaint by locating the button in the Toolbar labeled "Chief" and clicking on it.
In the dialog window that opens, type Patient reports waking at night short of breath.
When you have finished typing, click on the button labeled "Close the note form."

Step 4
Begin the visit by taking George's vital signs and medical history.
Use the form labeled "Vitals," which you will select from the Forms Manager.
Enter George's vital signs in the corresponding fields on the form as follows:

Temperature:	98.6
Respiration:	26
Pulse:	78
BP:	120/80
Height:	71
Weight:	175

When you have finished, check your work. If it is correct, proceed to step 5.

Step 5
Remain on the Forms tab. Take the patient's medical history by using the Short Intake form.
Locate and click on the button labeled "Forms" in the Toolbar at the top of your screen to invoke the Forms Manager window again.
Locate and click on the form labeled "Short Intake" as you have done in previous exercises.

226 Chapter 9 | Comprehensive Evaluation

Chapter 9 | Comprehensive Evaluation 227

◄ **COMPREHENSIVE EVALUATION** Learners will test their mastery of the material through a comprehensive evaluation found in Chapter 9 that includes a written exam and hands-on critical thinking exercise using the software.

Visualizing the Electronic Health Record

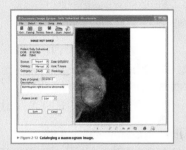

► Figure 2-12 **Cataloging a mammogram image.**

◄ ▼ ► **SCREEN CAPTURES** Easy-to-follow, step-by-step screen captures of the computer screens from the Medcin software illustrate the steps of the exercise. They serve as a ready reference to help learners orient themselves and assess their progress as they master content.

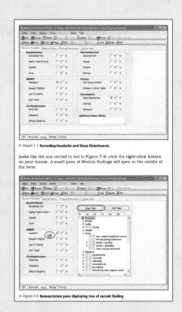

► Figure 7-7 **Recording Headache and Sleep Disturbances.**

looks like the one circled in red in Figure 7-8, click the **right-click button** on your mouse. A small pane of Medcin findings will open in the middle of the form.

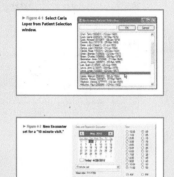

► Figure 6-15 **Prescription brand selection.**

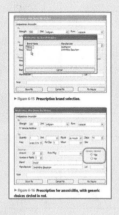

► Figure 4-1 **Select Carla Lopez from Patient Selection window.**

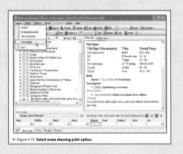

► Figure 4-15 **Select menu showing print option.**

► Figure 6-16 **Prescription for amoxicillin, with generic choices circled in red.**

► Figure 4-7 **New Encounter set for a "10 minute visit."**

► Figure 7-8 **Nomenclature pane displaying tree of current finding.**

► FIGURES AND TABLES

Illustrations and tables throughout help learners visualize workflow scenarios and technical concepts.

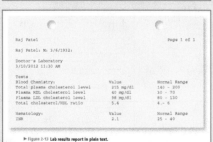

► Figure 1-4 **A healthcare professional enters data at patient's bedside.**

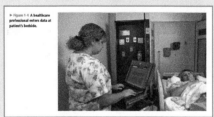

► Figure 2-13 **Lab results report in plain text.**

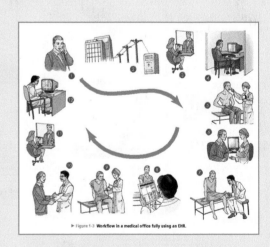

► Figure 1-3 **Workflow in a medical office fully using an EHR.**

The Medcin Student Edition Software

- Contains the entire Medcin nomenclature used in professional EHR systems. Medcin is the licensed core technology in many prominent EHR systems. Because the leading EHR systems for medical offices use the Medcin nomenclature as the technology underlying commercial EHR systems, students in most cases may apply skills they acquire in this course directly to an EHR application in their office. Those systems will not be identical to the student software, but they will seem very familiar to someone who has completed this course.
- Hands-on exercises are short, and have been designed to be completed in a normal class time.
- Multiuser software allows multiple students to work simultaneously, and keeps each student's work separate.
- All work is printed and no exercise requires saving. This allows students from multiple classes to share the same computer and avoids complications caused by saving and backing up databases. Printouts or file output from the exercises automatically include the student's login name or student ID.
- The printers will use the standard Windows system, and any compatible printer should work.
- For distance learning, the software allows the student to "print" to a file that will output the exercise document into a file in either PDF or XPS format. The output file can then be e-mailed or given to the instructor who may open and view the student's work with Adobe Reader or an ordinary web browser such as Microsoft Internet Explorer.
- All schools will receive Medcin Student Edition software they can install on the school network and computer lab workstations.

  Software may be installed in two ways: schools with networked computer labs can install a networked client/server system, or schools can install it locally on each student workstation.
- Students may download the individual workstation version and install it on their own (Windows-based) computer as well. This is ideal for distance learning students or those who wish to work outside the classroom.

Software Requirements

To complete the exercises in this book you will need access to the Medcin Student Edition software. If you are taking this course in a classroom, the software will already be installed. If you are in a distance learning program or working independently, you will need to download and install the software on a computer running the Windows operating system. Directions to download and install the software are found on the MyHealthProfessionsKit web page, which is described on the inside front cover of this book.

To complete the exercises in Chapter 2, you will also need access to the Internet and a web browser.

Minimum Workstation Requirements

Processor: 200 mHz Pentium

Operating system: Windows XP, Windows Vista, Windows 7 (or later)

RAM: 64 megabytes (free not counting OS)

Number of colors: 256 (8 bit color)

Display size (pixels per inch): 800 × 600 (1024 × 768 recommended)

Internet Explorer version 6 or later

Microsoft.Net Framework version 2.0 or later

You must have a mouse with at least two buttons that perform the right and left click functions.

Notice

The Medcin Student Edition software is licensed only for educational purposes, to allow the student to perform exercises in the textbook.

By using this program, a healthcare provider agrees that this product is not intended to suggest or replace any medical decisions or actions with respect to the patient's medical care and that the sole and exclusive responsibility for determining the accuracy, completeness, or appropriateness of any diagnostic, clinical, billing, or other medical information provided by the program and any underlying clinical database resides solely with the healthcare provider. Licensor assumes no responsibility for how such materials are used and disclaims all warranties, whether expressed or implied, including any warranty as to the quality, accuracy, or suitability of this information and product for any particular purpose.

About the Author

Richard Gartee is the author of seven college textbooks on health information technology, computerized medical systems, managed care, and electronic health records. Prior to becoming a full-time author and consultant, Richard spent 20 years in the design, development, and implementation of the preeminent practice management and electronic health records systems.

Richard also served as a liaison to other companies in the medical computer industry as well as Blue Cross/Blue Shield, a U.S. Department of Commerce International Trade Mission, and various universities.

Richard is a current or past member of many of the professional organizations and national standards groups recommended in this book:

◆ American Health Information Management Association (AHIMA)

◆ Healthcare Information Management Systems Society (HIMSS)

◆ American National Standards Institute (ANSI) X12n committee for development of electronic claims standards

◆ Health Level Seven (HL7) committee for development of claims attachment standards

◆ Workgroup for Electronic Data Interchange (WEDI) task force for development of electronic remittance guidelines

◆ A faculty member/speaker at the Medical Records Institute international Electronic Health Records Conference (TEPR) for 12 years.

Acknowledgments

This book was made possible by the contribution of many individuals and several of the most prominent commercial EHR vendors, whom I personally would like to thank and acknowledge here.

I first would like to thank Peter S. Goltra, David Lareau, and Roy Soltoff of Medicomp Systems, Inc. I am also indebted to the following commercial EHR vendors for allowing their copyrighted work to be reprinted herein. In alphabetical order:

Allscripts, LLC; McKesson, Inc.; Midmark Diagnostics Group; and **NextGen**.

The medical content and EHR theory of the textbook were greatly enhanced by my acquaintance with Dr. Allen R. Wenner, M.D., a physician, teacher, author, speaker, and expert on information technology, and with Dr. John Bachman, M.D., professor of family medicine at Mayo Clinic, Rochester, Minnesota.

Finally, I would like to acknowledge the help of all my editors who assisted me with this work, but especially Joan Gill, my executive editor. Thanks again, Joan!

I also would like to thank the academic reviewers, who took time to review and comment on this book.

Jane W. Dumas, MSN, CCMA, CHI
Allied Health Department Chair
Remington College–Cleveland West Campus
North Olmsted, OH

Christine Dzoga, CMA
MA Instructor
Illinois School of Health Careers
Chicago, IL

Alice Macomber
Medical Assisting University Program Chair
Keiser University–Port Saint Lucie Campus
Port St. Lucie, FL

Lane Miller, MBA/HCM
Director of Continuing Education
Medical Careers Institute, Virginia Beach Campus
Virginia Beach, VA

Marion D. Odom, NCMA
Medical Assisting Program Chair
Illinois School of Health Careers
Chicago, IL

Mary Warren-Oliver, B.S., CMRS
Medical Program Chair
Sanford-Brown College
Vienna, VA

Medcin Consulting Editors

Finally, I would like to recognize the work of the numerous doctors who consulted on the development of the Medcin nomenclature. These clinicians did not review the exercises in this book, but they did review the medical accuracy of the Medcin nomenclature that underlies this entire work. Therefore, I would like to acknowledge their work in the development and evolution of the knowledge base on which the Medcin Student Edition is based.

Medcin Consulting Editors

Robert G. Barone, M.D.
Clinical Assistant Professor of Ophthalmology
Cornell University Medical College;
Attending Surgeon, The New York Hospital
New York, NY

J. Gregory Cairncross, M.D.
Professor, Departments of Clinical Neurological Sciences and Oncology
University of Western Ontario and London Regional Cancer Centre
London, Ontario, Canada

Richard P. Cohen, M.D.
Clinical Associate Professor of Medicine
Cornell University Medical College;
Associate Attending Physician, The New York Hospital
New York, NY

Bradley A. Connor, M.D.
Clinical Assistant Professor of Medicine
Cornell University Medical College;
Adjunct Faculty, Rockefeller University;
Assistant Attending Physician, The New York Hospital
New York, NY

David R. Gastfriend, M.D.
Assistant Professor in Psychiatry
Harvard Medical School;
Director of Addiction Services
Massachusetts General Hospital
Boston, MA

Stephanie M. Heidelberg, M.D.
Medical Director, Adult, Older Adult Programs
American Day Treatment Centers, Fairfax, VA;
Psychiatrist, Adult Day Treatment Program,
Northwest Mental Health Center, Reston, VA

Edmund M. Herrold, M.D., Ph.D.
Associate Professor of Medicine
Director, Section of Biophysics and Biomechanics
Division of Cardiovascular Pathophysiology
Cornell University Medical College;
Associate Attending Physician, The New York Hospital
New York, NY

Allan N. Houghton, M.D.
Professor of Medicine and Immunology
Cornell University Medical College;
Chair, Immunology Program,
Memorial Sloan-Kettering Cancer Center
New York, NY

Ralph H. Hruban, M.D.
Associate Professor of Pathology
Associate Professor of Oncology
The Johns Hopkins School of Medicine;
Director, Division of Cardiovascular-Respiratory Pathology
The Johns Hopkins Hospital
Baltimore, MD

Mark Lachs, M.D., MPH
Assistant Professor of Medicine
Cornell University Medical College;
Chief, Geriatrics Unit, Department of Medicine
The New York Hospital
New York, NY

Fredrick A. McCurdy, M.D., Ph.D.
Associate Professor of Pediatrics
Director of Pediatric Undergraduate Education
University of Nebraska College of Medicine
Omaha, NE

Paul F. Miskovitz, M.D.
Clinical Associate Professor of Medicine
Cornell University Medical College;
Associate Attending Physician
The New York Hospital, New York, NY

Preeti Pancholi, Ph.D.
Staff Scientist, Department of Virology and Parasitology
Kimball Research Institute
New York Blood Center
New York, NY

Louis N. Pangaro, M.D.
Associate Professor, Clinical Medicine
Vice Chairman for Educational Programs,
Department of Medicine, Uniformed Services
University of The Health Sciences,
F. Edward Herbert School of Medicine
Bethesda, MD

Edward J. Parrish, M.D., M.S.
Assistant Professor of Medicine
Cornell University Medical College;
Department of Medicine, Division of Rheumatology,
The New York Hospital, Hospital for Special Surgery
New York, NY

William B. Patterson, M.D., MPH
Assistant Professor of Environmental Health
Boston University School of Public Health
Boston, MA;
President, New England Health Center
Wilmington, MA

David Posnett, M.D.
Associate Professor of Medicine
Cornell University Medical College;
Division of Immunology, Department of Medicine
The New York Hospital, New York, NY

Calvin W. Roberts, M.D.
Professor of Ophthalmology,
Cornell University Medical College
New York, NY

Ronald C. Silvestri, M.D.
Assistant Professor of Medicine
Harvard Medical School;
Director, Medical Intensive Care Unit
Deaconess Hospital
Boston, MA

Michael Thorpe, M.D.
Musculoskeletal Radiology Fellow
The Hospital for Special Surgery
New York, NY

Anshu Vashishtha, M.D., Ph.D.
Adjunct Faculty Member
Laboratory of Bacterial Pathogenesis and Immunology
The Rockefeller University;
Clinical Fellow in Allergy and Immunology,
The New York Hospital, New York, NY

H. Hallett Whitman, III, M.D.
Clinical Assistant Professor of Medicine
Cornell University Medical College;
Clinical Affiliate, Hypertension Center
The New York Hospital, New York, NY;
Attending Physician in Internal Medicine and
Rheumatology
Summit Medical Group, Summit, NJ

E. David Wright, M.D.
Clinical Assistant Professor of Medicine
Department of Dermatology
University of Virginia Health Sciences Center
Charlottesville, VA;
Dermatology Associates, Inc.;
Attending Physician, Winchester Medical Center
Winchester, VA

Joseph Zibrak, M.D.
Assistant Professor of Medicine
Harvard Medical School;
Associate Chief of Pulmonary and Critical Care Medicine
Beth Israel Deaconess Medical Center
Boston, MA

Electronic Health Records— An Overview

Learning Outcomes

After completing this chapter, you should be able to:

◆ Define electronic health records

◆ Understand the core functions of an electronic health record as defined by the Institute of Medicine

◆ Explain why electronic health records are important

◆ Discuss social forces that are driving the adoption of electronic health records

◆ Describe the flow of medical information into the chart

◆ Compare the workflow of an office using paper charts to that of an office using electronic health records

◆ Explain why patient visits should be documented at the point of care

Evolution of Electronic Health Records

The idea of computerizing patients' medical records has been around for more than 30 years, but only in the past decade has it become widely adopted. Prior to the electronic health record (EHR), a patient's medical records consisted of handwritten notes, typed reports, and test results, all of which were stored in a paper file system. Although paper medical records are still used today in many healthcare facilities, the transition to electronic health records is under way.

Beginning in 1991, the IOM (which stands for the Institute of Medicine of the National Academies) sponsored studies and created reports that led the way toward the concepts we have in place today for electronic health records. Originally, the IOM called them *computer-based patient records*.[1] During its evolution, the EHR has had many other names including electronic medical records, computerized medical records, longitudinal patient records, and electronic charts. All of these names referred to essentially the same thing, which in 2003, the IOM renamed as the electronic health record or EHR.

Institute of Medicine

An Institute of Medicine (IOM) report[2] put forth a set of eight core functions that an EHR should be capable of performing:

Health Information and Data An EHR should provide a defined data set that includes such items as medical and nursing diagnoses, a medication list, allergies, demographics, clinical narratives, and laboratory test results. It should also provide improved access to information needed by care providers when they need it.

Results Management With an EHR, providers can access the results of computerized reports more easily than paper reports whenever and wherever needed.

◆ The reduced lag time allows for quicker recognition and treatment of medical problems.

◆ The automated display of previous test results makes it possible to reduce redundancy and avoid additional testing.

◆ The use of electronic results allows for better interpretation and easier detection of abnormalities, thereby ensuring appropriate follow-up.

◆ Access to electronic consults and patient consents can establish critical links and improve care coordination among multiple providers, as well as between provider and patient.

Order Management Computerized provider order entry (CPOE) systems can improve workflow processes by eliminating lost orders and the ambiguities caused by illegible handwriting, generating related orders automatically, monitoring for duplicate orders, and reducing the time required to fill orders.

◆ CPOE systems for medications reduce the number of errors in medication dose and frequency, drug allergies, and drug–drug interactions.

◆ The use of CPOE, in conjunction with an EHR, also improves clinician productivity.

Decision Support Computerized decision support systems help healthcare providers manage issues of prevention, diagnosis, and management; drug

---

[1]R. S. Dick and E. B. Steen, *The Computer-based Patient Record: An Essential Technology for Health Care* (Washington, DC: Institute of Medicine, National Academies Press, 1991, revised 1997, 2000).
[2]Section based on material in Dick and Steen, *The Computer-based Patient Record.*

prescriptions and adverse interactions; and detection of adverse events and disease outbreaks.

◆ Computerized reminders and prompts improve preventive practices in areas such as vaccinations, breast cancer screening, colorectal screening, and cardiovascular risk reduction.

Electronic Communication and Connectivity Electronic communication among care partners can enhance patient safety and quality of care, especially for patients who have multiple providers in multiple settings that must coordinate care plans.

◆ Electronic connectivity is essential in creating and populating EHR systems with data from laboratories, pharmacies, radiology departments, and other providers.

◆ Secure e-mail and web messaging have been shown to be effective in facilitating communication among providers and with patients, thus allowing for greater continuity of care and more timely interventions.

◆ Automatic alerts to providers regarding abnormal laboratory results reduce the time until an appropriate treatment is ordered.

◆ Electronic communication is fundamental to the creation of an integrated health record, both within a setting and across settings and institutions.

Patient Support Computer-based patient education has been found to be successful in improving control of chronic illnesses, such as diabetes, in primary care.

◆ Patients can use electronic devices to conduct home monitoring. Examples include self-testing by patients with asthma (spirometry), glucose monitors for patients with diabetes, and Holter monitors for patients with heart conditions. Data from monitoring devices can be merged into the EHR, as shown in Figure 1-1.

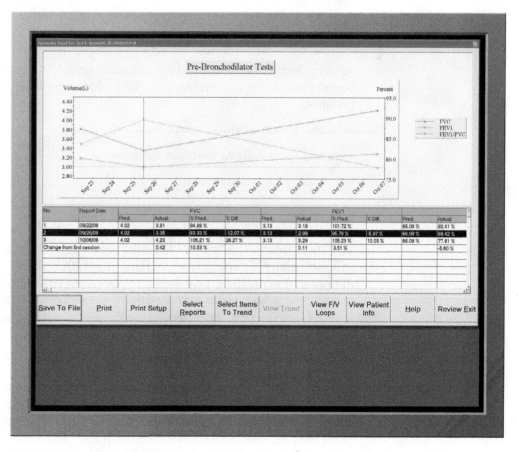

Courtesy of Midmark Diagnostics Group.

▶ Figure 1-1 **Data from digital spirometer transfers to EHR.**

Administrative Processes and Reporting Electronic scheduling systems increase the efficiency of healthcare organizations and provide better, timelier service to patients.

◆ Communication and content standards are important in the billing and claims management area.

◆ Electronic authorization and prior approvals can eliminate delays and confusion; immediate validation of insurance eligibility results in more timely payments and less paperwork.

◆ EHR data can be analyzed to identify patients who are potentially eligible for clinical trials, as well as candidates for chronic disease management programs.

◆ Reporting tools support drug recalls.

Reporting and Population Health Public- and private-sector reporting requirements at the federal, state, and local levels for patient safety and quality, as well as for public health, are more easily met with computerized data.

◆ EHRs eliminate the labor-intensive and time-consuming abstraction of data from paper records and the errors that often occur in a manual process.

◆ They facilitate the reporting of key quality indicators used for the internal quality improvement efforts of many healthcare organizations.

◆ They also improve public health surveillance and timely reporting of adverse reactions and disease outbreaks.

In addition to the IOM, ideas from the Computer-based Patient Record Institute and the Health Insurance Portability and Accountability Act help us define the EHR.

Computer-based Patient Record Institute

Another early contributor to the thinking on EHR systems was the Computer-based Patient Record Institute (CPRI), which identified three key criteria for an EHR:

◆ Capture data at the point of care.

◆ Integrate data from multiple sources.

◆ Provide decision support.

Health Insurance Portability and Accountability Act

The 1996 Health Insurance Portability and Accountability Act (HIPAA) Privacy Rule strengthened the privacy of patient health records. The HIPAA Security Rule did not define an EHR, but seemed to broaden the definition. The Security Rule established protection for *all* personally identifiable health information stored in an electronic format. Thus, everything about a patient stored in a healthcare provider's system is protected and treated as part of the patient's EHR.

EHR Defined

In *Electronic Health Records: Changing the Vision*, authors Murphy, Waters, Hanken, and Pfeiffer define the EHR to include "any information relating to the past, present or future physical/mental health, or condition of an individual which resides in electronic system(s) used to capture, transmit, receive, store, retrieve, link and manipulate multimedia data for the primary purpose of providing health care and health-related services."[3] EHRs can include dental health records as well.

The core functions defined by the IOM and CPRI suggest that the EHR is not just a repository for stored data, but also encompasses what can be done with that data. In the broadest sense, *electronic health records are the portions of a patient's medical records that are stored in a computer system as well as the functional benefits derived from having an electronic health record.*

Social Forces Driving EHR Adoption

Visionary leaders in medical informatics have been making the case for the EHR for a long time. However, the combination of several important reports caught the public's attention and set in motion economic and political forces that are driving the transformation of our medical records systems.

Health Safety The IOM published a report stating:

> Health care in the United States is not as safe as it should be—and can be. At least 44,000 people, and perhaps as many as 98,000 people, die in hospitals each year as a result of medical errors that could have been prevented, according to estimates from two major studies.
>
> Beyond their cost in human lives, preventable medical errors exact other significant tolls. They have been estimated to result in total costs (including the expense of additional care necessitated by the errors, lost income and household productivity, and disability) of between $17 billion and $29 billion per year in hospitals nation-wide. Errors also are costly in terms of loss of trust in the healthcare system by patients and diminished satisfaction by both patients and health professionals.
>
> A variety of factors have contributed to the nation's epidemic of medical errors. One oft-cited problem arises from the decentralized and fragmented nature of the healthcare delivery system—or "non-system" to some observers. When patients see multiple providers in different settings, none of whom has access to complete information, it becomes easier for things to go wrong.[4]

These statements got the attention of the press and public. They also got the attention of 150 of the nation's largest employers.

Health Costs Employers who sponsored employee health insurance programs had become frustrated by the increasing costs of health insurance benefits and the fact that they had little or no say about the quality of care provided by those benefits. Following the release of the IOM report just discussed, these employers formed the Leapfrog group. Leapfrog created a strategy that tied the purchase of group health insurance benefits to quality care standards.

Leapfrog also promoted CPOE as a means of reducing errors, in part because of a study by the Center for Information Technology Leadership that found more than 130,000 life-threatening situations caused by adverse drug reactions alone. The study suggested that $44 billion could be saved annually by installing CPOE systems in ambulatory settings.

---

[3]Gretchen Murphy, Kathleen Waters, Mary A. Hanken, and Maureen Pfeiffer, eds., *Electronic Health Records: Changing the Vision* (Philadelphia: W. B. Saunders Company, 1999), 5.

[4]Linda T. Kohn, Janet M. Corrigan, and Molla S. Donaldson, eds., *To Err Is Human: Building a Safer Health System* (Washington, DC: Committee on Quality of Health Care in America, Institute of Medicine, 1999).

Government Response The government and private sector responses to the IOM report were swift and positive. Almost immediately, President Bill Clinton's administration issued an executive order instructing government agencies that conduct or oversee healthcare programs to implement proven techniques for reducing medical errors, and creating a task force to find new strategies for reducing errors. Congress appropriated $50 million to the Agency for Healthcare Research and Quality (AHRQ) to support a variety of efforts targeted at reducing medical errors.

President George W. Bush followed through by establishing the Office of the National Coordinator for Health Information Technology (ONC) under the U.S. Department of Health and Human Services (HHS) to "develop, maintain, and direct the implementation of a strategic plan to guide the nationwide implementation of interoperable health information technology in both the public and private healthcare sectors that will reduce medical errors, improve quality, and produce greater value for healthcare expenditures."[5]

More recently, President Barack Obama identified the EHR as a priority for his administration and signed into law the Health Information Technology for Economic and Clinical Health (HITECH) Act. The act promotes the widespread adoption of EHRs and authorizes Medicare incentive payments to doctors and hospitals using a certified EHR and eventually implements financial penalties for physicians and hospitals that do not use one.[6]

Changing Society

Changes in the way we live have also made paper medical records outdated. In an increasingly mobile society, patients relocate and change doctors more frequently than in the past and thus need to transfer their medical records from previous doctors to new ones. Additionally, many patients no longer have a single general practitioner who provides their total care. Increased specialization and the development of new methods of diagnostic and preventive medicine require the ability to share exam records among different specialists and testing facilities.

The Internet, one of the strongest forces for social change in the past decade, also affects healthcare. Consumers are becoming accustomed to being able to access very sensitive information securely over the web. They are beginning to ask "Why can't I access my health records online?" Additionally, there are literally millions of health-related pieces of information on the web. Patients are arriving at their doctor's office armed with questions and sometimes answers. Medical information previously unavailable to the average consumer is now as easy to access as searching Google™ or WebMD®.

Critical Thinking Exercise 1: EHR News

1. The topic of electronic health records is frequently in the news. Describe something you have read or seen on TV or on the Internet about electronic health records.

---

[5]President George W. Bush, Executive Order #13335, April 27, 2004.

[6]H.R. 1 American Recovery and Reinvestment Act of 2009, Title XIII Health Information Technology for Economic and Clinical Health, February 17, 2009.

Flow of Medical Information into the Patient Chart

Whether medical records are paper or electronic, the clinician's exam notes are usually documented in a defined structure organized into four components:

◆ Subjective

◆ Objective

◆ Assessment

◆ Plan

Charts in this format are referred to as SOAP notes. The acronym represents the first letter of the words subjective, objective, assessment, and plan. Later in this book, exercises using EHR software will follow the SOAP format.

Historically, a patient's medical records consisted of handwritten notes, typed reports, and test results stored in a paper file system. A separate file folder was created and stored at each location where the patient was examined or treated. X-ray films and other radiology records typically were stored separately from the chart, even when they were created at the same medical facility.

These are some of the drawbacks to paper records: Handwritten records often are abbreviated, cryptic, or illegible. When information is to be used by another medical practice, the charts must be copied and faxed or mailed to the other office. Even in one practice with multiple locations, the chart must be transported from one office to another when a patient is seen at a different location than usual. Paper records are not easily searchable. For example, if a practice is notified that all patients on a particular drug need to be contacted, the only way to find those patients is by literally opening every chart and looking at the medications lists.

Certainly, improved legibility and the ability to find, share, and search patient records are strong points for an EHR. EHRs also have additional benefits that take the practice of medicine to levels that cannot be achieved with paper records. Four examples of this are trend analysis, alerts, health maintenance, and decision support. These will be covered in more detail in Chapter 2.

However, the EHR requires not only computers and software, but also changes in the way providers work. To understand this, let us compare the workflow in a medical office using paper charts with a medical office using an EHR system.

Workflow of an Office Using Paper Charts

Follow the arrows in Figure 1-2 as you read the following description of a workflow in a primary care medical practice using paper charts.

1 An established patient phones the doctor's office and schedules an appointment.

2 The night before the appointment, the patient charts are pulled from the medical record filing system and organized for the next day's patients.

3 On the day of the appointment, the patient arrives at the office and is asked to confirm that insurance and demographic information on file is correct.

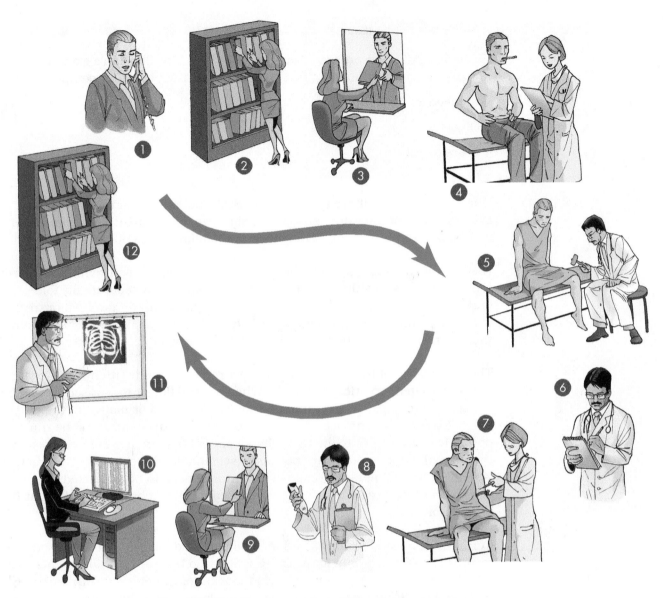

▶ Figure 1-2 **Workflow in a medical office using paper charts.**

The patient is given a clipboard with a blank medical history form and asked to complete it. The form asks the reason for today's visit and asks the patient to report any previous history, any changes to medications, new allergies, and so on.

④ Patient is moved to an exam room and is asked to wait. A healthcare professional takes vital signs, reviews the form the patient completed, and may ask for more details about the reason for the visit, which usually is called the "chief complaint." The healthcare professional writes down the vital signs and chief complaint on a form that is placed at the front of the chart along with the updated patient form.

Depending on the reason for the visit, the patient may be asked to undress, in which case the healthcare professional will leave the room while the patient does so.

⑤ The clinician (doctor or other healthcare provider) enters the exam room and discusses the reason for the visit and reviews the symptoms.

Subjective—The patient is asked to describe in his or her own words what the problem is, what the symptoms are, and what he or she is experiencing.

Objective—The clinician performs a physical exam and makes observations about what he or she finds.

Assessment—Applying his or her training to the subjective and objective findings, the clinician arrives at a decision of what might be the cause of the patient's condition or what further tests might be necessary.

Plan of Treatment—The clinician prescribes a treatment, medication, or orders further tests. Perhaps a follow-up visit at a later date is recommended. A note will be made in the chart of each element of the plan.

6 If medications have been ordered, a handwritten prescription will be given to the patient or phoned to the pharmacy. A note of the prescription will be written in the patient's chart.

The provider marks one or more billing codes and one or more diagnosis codes on the chart and leaves the exam room.

7 If lab work has been ordered, a medical assistant will obtain the necessary specimen and send the order to the lab.

8 At many practices, the physician creates the exam note from memory, either handwriting in the chart or dictating the subjective, objective, assessment, and plan of treatment information.

9 When the patient is dressed, the patient will be escorted to the checkout area. The healthcare professional or staff may give the patient education material or medication instructions.

If x-rays or other diagnostic tests have been ordered at another facility, the office staff may call on behalf of the patient and schedule the tests.

If a follow-up visit has been indicated, the patient will be scheduled for the next appointment.

10 The dictated notes are later transcribed and returned to the doctor to review before being permanently stored in the chart.

11 If lab, x-ray, or other diagnostic tests have been ordered, the results and reports are subsequently sent to the practice either by fax or on paper a number of days later. When received, they are filed in the patient's chart and the chart is sent to the clinician for review. After review, the reports are filed in the paper chart.

12 The paper chart is filed again. Note that the chart may have to be refiled and pulled each time a new document, such as the transcription or lab report, is added.

One obvious downside to paper charts is accessibility. If the patient chart is needed for a follow-up visit or by another provider, the timing may be such that the chart has not been returned to the file room because it is pending dictation or the provider is reviewing test results.

Workflow of an Office Fully Using an EHR

Follow the arrows in Figure 1-3 as you read the following description of a workflow of a patient visit to an office that fully uses the electronic capabilities that

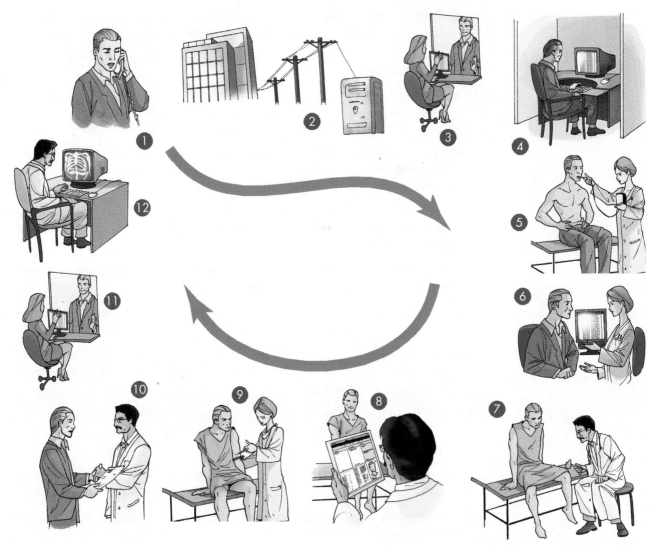

▶ Figure 1-3 **Workflow in a medical office fully using an EHR.**

are available in EHR systems today, including patient participation in the process and the capabilities of the Internet.

① An established patient phones the doctor's office and schedules an appointment.

Internet Alternative: Patients are increasingly able to request an appointment and receive a confirmation via the Internet.

② The night before the appointment, the medical office computer electronically verifies insurance eligibility for patients scheduled the next day.

③ On the day of the appointment, the patient arrives at the office and is asked to confirm that the demographic information on file is still correct.

④ A receptionist or medical assistant asks the patient to complete a medical history and reason for today's visit using a computer in a private area of the waiting room. The patient completes a computer-guided questionnaire concerning his or her symptoms and medical history.

Internet Alternative: Some medical practices allow patients to use the Internet to complete the history and symptom questionnaire before coming to the office.

⑤ When the patient has completed the questionnaire, the system alerts a healthcare professional that the patient is ready to move to an exam room.

The healthcare professional measures the patient's height and weight and records it in the EHR. Using a modern device, vital signs for blood pressure, temperature, and pulse are recorded and wirelessly transferred into the EHR.

⑥ **Subjective**—The healthcare professional and patient review the patient-entered symptoms and history. Where necessary the healthcare professional edits the record to add clarification or refinement.

⑦ The physician enters the exam room and discusses the reason for the visit and reviews with the patient the information already in the chart.

Objective—The clinician performs the physical exam. The clinician typically makes a mental provisional diagnosis. This is used to select a list or template of findings to quickly document the physical exam in the EHR.

The EHR presents a list of problems the patient reported in past visits that have not been resolved. The physician reviews each, examining additional body systems as necessary, and marks the improvement, worsening, or resolution of each problem.

Assessment—Applying his or her training to the subjective and objective findings, the clinician arrives at a decision of one or more diagnoses, and decides if further tests might be warranted.

⑧ **Plan of Treatment**—The clinician prescribes a treatment, medication, and/or orders further tests using the EHR.

If medication is to be ordered, the physician writes the prescription electronically. The prescription is compared to the patient's allergy records and current drugs. The physician is advised if there are any contraindications or potential problems. The prescription is compared to the formulary of drugs covered by the patient's insurance plan and the physician is advised if an alternate drug is recommended (thereby avoiding a subsequent phone call from the pharmacist to revise the prescription). The prescription is then transmitted directly to the patient's pharmacy.

A built-in function of the EHR accurately calculates the correct evaluation and management code used for billing. The billing code is confirmed by the physician and automatically transferred to the billing system.

When the visit is complete, so is the exam note. The physician signs the note electronically at the conclusion of the visit.

⑨ If lab work has been ordered, a medical assistant will obtain the necessary specimen and send the order electronically to the lab.

⑩ **Patient Education**—Because of the efficiency of the EHR system, the physician has more personal time with the patient for counseling or patient education. In many systems the provider can display and annotate pictures of body areas for patient education, and print them so that the patient can take them home.

When the patient is dressed, he or she is given patient education material, medication instructions, and a copy of the exam notes from the current visit. Allowing the patient to take away a written record of the visit enables better compliance with the doctor's plan of care and recommended treatments.

⑪ The patient is escorted to the checkout area.

If x-rays or other diagnostic tests have been ordered at another facility, the office staff may call on behalf of the patient and schedule the tests.

If a follow-up visit has been indicated, the patient will be scheduled for the next appointment.

⑫ If lab tests were ordered, the results are sent to the doctor electronically, are reviewed on screen, and automatically merged into the EHR.

If radiology or other diagnostic reports are sent to the practice electronically as text reports, they are imported into the EHR and can be reviewed by the physician online.

Accessibility is not a problem in the EHR system because there is no chart to "refile." Multiple providers can access the patient's chart, even simultaneously; for example, a physician could review the previous lab results before entering the exam room, even if a medical assistant is concurrently recording vital signs in the chart.

Critical Thinking Exercise 2: Think about Workflow

Having compared the two workflow scenarios, we see the immediate advantages of the EHR for both the patient and clinician. Think about the workflow of the office that used paper charts (refer to Figure 1-2 if necessary.) Answer the following questions about the first workflow:

1. What was the medical assistant or other healthcare professional doing at the time of the patient interaction?

2. Could that person have recorded this data in a computer?

3. Could that person have saved time later?

4. Could the data be entered by someone other than the person seeing the patient?

The patient completed a form concerning any previous history, any changes to medications, new allergies, and so on.

5. Could the patient have used a computer, or could the form have been designed to be read by a computer?

6. Could the patient have completed the information before the visit?

The medical assistant recorded various health measurements (vital signs) in the exam room.

7. Could the healthcare professional have recorded the "chief complaint" or the vital signs in a computer instead of on a paper chart?

8. Were any of the instruments used capable of transferring their measurements to a computer system?

During the physical exam, the physician made observations and an assessment. This was later dictated from memory, subsequently transcribed by a typist, and finally reviewed and signed by the physician.

9. Is the time it would take to record the observations and assessment in a computer comparable to the time it takes to dictate and review the notes later?

The physician prescribed medications and ordered tests.

10. Would the time spent entering the prescriptions on a computer justify the benefits of electronic prescribing?

11. Are electronic results available from the laboratories the medical practice uses?

12. Would ordering a test electronically improve the matching of results to orders when the tests were completed?

Documenting at the Point of Care

A goal of using an EHR system is to improve the accuracy and completeness of the patient record. One way to achieve this is to record the information in the EHR at the time it is happening. This is called *point-of-care documentation*. In a physician's office, this means completing the SOAP note before the patient ever leaves the office. In an inpatient setting, this means that healthcare professionals enter vital signs and notes about the patient at bedside, not at the end of their shift. Figure 1-4 shows a healthcare professional entering data while with the patient.

▶ Figure 1-4 **A healthcare professional enters data at patient's bedside.**

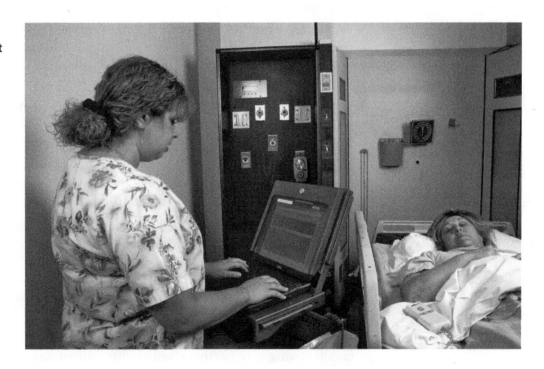

Leading physician experts on the EHR, Allen R. Wenner, an M.D. in Columbia, South Carolina, and John W. Bachman, an M.D. at the Mayo Clinic, wrote:

> Documenting an encounter at the point of care is the most efficient method of practicing medicine because the physician completes the medical record at the time of a patient's visit. Dictation time is saved and the need for personal dictation aides is eliminated. Thus, point-of-care documentation is less expensive than traditional dictation with its associated high cost of transcription. In addition, the physician can sign the note immediately.
>
> Patient care is improved because the patient can leave with a complete copy of the medical record, a step that stimulates compliance. The delivery process is improved

with point-of-care documentation because referrals can be accomplished with full information available at the time that the referral is needed. For these benefits to occur, the clinical workflow changes to improve efficiency, increase data accuracy, and lower the overall cost of healthcare delivery.[7]

The EHR system strives to improve patient healthcare by giving the provider and patient access to complete, up-to-date records of past and present conditions; it also enables the records to be used in ways that paper medical records could not. The sooner the data is entered, the sooner it is available for other providers and the patient. Chapters 3 through 8 will explore how data is entered in the EHR and focus on ways EHR systems speed up data entry, enabling clinicians to achieve point-of-care documentation in real time.

Chapter One Summary

Electronic health records are the portions of a patient's medical records that are stored in a computer system as well as the functional benefits derived from having an electronic health record.

The IOM set forth eight core functions that an EHR should be capable of performing:

◆ **Health information and data** Provide improved access to information needed by care providers by using a defined data set that includes medical and nursing diagnoses, a medication list, allergies, demographics, clinical narratives, laboratory test results, and more.

◆ **Results management** The use of EHRs leads to quicker recognition and better interpretation and treatment of medical problems. They also reduce redundant testing and improve care coordination among multiple providers.

◆ **Order management** CPOE systems improve workflow, eliminate lost orders and ambiguities caused by illegible handwriting, monitor for duplicate orders, and reduce the time required to fill orders.

◆ **Decision support** Computerized decision support systems help healthcare providers with diagnosis, and disease management; drug prescriptions; and detection of adverse events and disease outbreaks. Computerized reminders and prompts improve preventive practices in areas such as vaccinations, breast cancer screening, colorectal screening, and cardiovascular risk reduction.

◆ **Electronic communication and connectivity** EHRs help improve communication among care partners, enhancing patient safety and quality of care, especially for patients who have multiple providers.

◆ **Patient support** Patients benefit from patient education and the ability to do home monitoring via electronic devices.

◆ **Administrative processes and reporting** EHRs increase the efficiency of healthcare organizations and provide better, timelier service to patients.

---

[7]Allen R. Wenner and John W. Bachman, "Transforming the Physician Practice: Interviewing Patients with a Computer," Chap. 26 in *Healthcare Information Management Systems: Cases, Strategies, and Solutions*, 3rd ed., ed. Marion J. Ball, Charlotte A. Weaver, and Joan M. Kiel (New York: Springer Science+Business Media, Inc., 2004), 297–319. Copyright © 2004 Springer Science+Business Media, Inc., New York.

◆ **Reporting and population health** EHRs facilitate the reporting of key quality indicators and timely reporting of adverse reactions and disease outbreaks.

The CPRI identified three key criteria for an EHR:

◆ Capture data at the point of care.

◆ Integrate data from multiple sources.

◆ Provide decision support.

A patient encounter document is organized into four components:

◆ Subjective

◆ Objective

◆ Assessment

◆ Plan.

The EHR systems strive to improve patient healthcare by giving the provider and patient access to complete, up-to-date records of past and present conditions.

Documenting at the point of care refers to healthcare providers recording their findings at the time of the encounter, not after they have left the patient.

Testing Your Knowledge of Chapter 1

1. What does the acronym EHR stand for?
2. What is the definition of an EHR?
3. Explain the benefits of EHR over paper charts.
4. List the eight core functions that an EHR should be capable of performing.
5. List the three criteria of an EHR defined by CPRI.
6. What are the four defined sections in a SOAP note?
7. Why are electronic health records important?
8. Describe what generally takes place from the time a patient checks in at a physician's office until the patient checks out.
9. Describe what points in the workflow are different between offices using a paper chart and those using an electronic chart.
10. Explain why patient visits should be documented at the point of care.
11. Name at least three forces driving the change to EHRs.
12. What does the acronym CPOE stand for?
13. How does the HITECH act promote EHR adoption?
14. What is one benefit of giving the patient a copy of the completed encounter note at the end of the visit?
15. What three benefits of electronic results were identified by the IOM report?

2

Functional EHR Systems

Learning Outcomes

After completing this chapter, you should be able to:

- Explain how the format of EHR data determines functional benefits

- Compare different EHR data formats

- Discuss the limitations of certain types of data

- Describe the importance of codified electronic health records

- Have an understanding of prominent EHR code sets such as SNOMED-CT, MEDCIN, and LOINC

- Name different methods of capturing and recording EHR data

- Describe the functional benefits derived from using an EHR

- Provide examples of the EHR functions of trend analysis, alerts, health maintenance, and decision support

Format of Data Determines Potential Benefits

The ability to easily find, share, and search patient records makes an EHR superior to a paper record system. However, remember that Chapter 1 defined the EHR as the portions of the patient's medical record stored in the computer system *as well as the functional benefits derived from them.*

In Chapter 1 we discussed eight core functions defined by the IOM that an EHR should be capable of performing. Four of the *functional benefits* identified by the IOM are health maintenance, trend analysis, alerts, and decision support. The form in which the data is stored determines to what extent the computer can use the content of the EHR to provide additional functions that improve the quality of care.

This chapter examines the forms in which EHR data is stored, explores how functional benefits are derived from it, and explains how data are entered.

EHR Data Formats

The various ways in which medical records data are stored in the database may be broadly categorized into three forms, as discussed next.

Digital Images EHR data can include digital images. Digital images can be retrieved and displayed by the computer, but a human is required to interpret the meaning of the content. This category may be subcategorized as follows:

Diagnostic Images such as digital x-rays, CAT scans, digital pathology reports, and even annotated drawings

Scanned Documents such as paper forms, old medical records, letters, or even sound files of dictated notes.

Text Files The second type of data, text files, includes word processing files of transcribed exam notes and also text reports. It is principally obtained in the EHR by importing text files from outside sources.

Discrete Data This third form of stored information in an EHR, discrete data, is the easiest for the computer to use. It can be instantly searched, retrieved, and combined or reported in different ways. Discrete data in an EHR may be subcategorized as follows:

Fielded Data in which each piece of information is assigned its own position in a computer record called a *field*. The meaning of the information is inferred from its position in the record. For example, a record of a patient's medical problem might look like this:

"knee injury","20120331","improved","20120427"

The fields in this example are surrounded by quotation marks. The computer would be programmed to look for the name of the problem in the first field, the date of onset in the second field, the status of the problem in the third field, and the date of the last exam in the fourth field.

Coded Data is fielded data that also contains codes in addition to or in place of descriptive text. Codes eliminate ambiguities about the clinician's meaning.

A codified EHR record of the same knee problem might look like this:

"8442", "knee injury","20120331","improved","20120427"

Limitations of Certain Types of Data

An EHR offers improved accessibility to patient records over a paper chart. That is certainly a functional benefit of any EHR regardless of the format of its data. However, to achieve its full functional benefits, the computer must be able to quickly and accurately identify the information contained within the records.

As mentioned earlier, digital image data can be retrieved and displayed by the computer, but a human is required to interpret the meaning of the content. While this is beneficial for sharing diagnostic images, if the bulk of the EHR is simply scanned paper documents only one or two of the IOM criteria defined in Chapter 1 are satisfied.

Healthcare professionals can read any text data that is entered; additionally, that data can also be searched by the computer for research purposes. However, text data is seldom used for generating alerts, trend analysis, decision support, or other real-time EHR functions, because the search capability is slow and the results often ambiguous.

Fielded data is the most common way to store information in computers and EHR systems. It is fast and efficient and uses very little storage space. However, unless the fielded data is also codified, the meaning of the data can be ambiguous.

Within medicine, many different terms are used to describe the same symptom, condition, or observation. Additionally, clinicians often use short abbreviations to document their observations in a patient chart. This makes it difficult for a computer to compare notes from one physician to another. For example providers at two different clinics might record a knee injury problem differently:

Dr. 1: "twisted his knee"

Dr. 2: "knee sprain."

A search of medical records by the description "knee injury" might not find the records created by either clinician.

Coded data is the term used to describe data that are stored with a code in the medical record in addition to the text description. Such a record is considered a *codified record*. The benefit of using codified records is that the EHR system can instantly find and match the desired information by code regardless of the clinician's choice of words. A codified EHR is more useful than a text-based record because it precisely identifies the clinician's finding or treatment.

EHR data stored in a fielded, codified form adds significant value, but if the codes are not standard it will be difficult to exchange medical record data between different EHR systems or facilities. Remember, the exchange of data is one of the eight core functions defined by the IOM. Using a national standard code set instead of proprietary codes to codify the data will better enable the exchange of medical records among systems, improve the accuracy of the content, and open the door to the other functional benefits derived from having an electronic health record.

Standard EHR Coding Systems

EHR coding systems are called *nomenclatures*. EHR nomenclatures differ from other code sets and classification systems in that they are designed to codify the details and nuance of the patient–clinician encounter. EHR nomenclatures are different from billing code sets in this respect. For example, a procedure code used for billing an office visit does not describe what the clinician observed about the patient during the visit, just the type of visit and complexity of the exam. EHR nomenclatures need to have a lot more codes to describe the details of the exam; for this reason, they are said to be more *granular*. Two prominent nomenclatures for EHR records are SNOMED-CT® and MEDCIN®. Another prominent coding system, LOINC®, is used for lab results.

Unfortunately, many hospital systems use none of these standard systems, having instead developed internal coding schemes applicable only to their facilities. These internal systems function within the organization, but create problems when trying to integrate other software or exchange data within a regional health information organization (RHIO). RHIOs are discussed later in this chapter.

SNOMED-CT

SNOMED stands for Systematized Nomenclature of Medicine; CT stands for Clinical Terms. SNOMED-CT is a medical nomenclature developed by the College of American Pathologists and the United Kingdom's National Health Service. It is a merger of two previous coding systems, SNOMED and the Read codes.

MEDCIN

MEDCIN is a medical nomenclature and knowledge base developed by Medicomp Systems, Inc., in collaboration with physicians on staff at the Cornell, Harvard, Johns Hopkins, and other major medical centers. The purpose of the MEDCIN nomenclature and the intent of the design differentiate it from other coding standards. For example, whereas SNOMED-CT and other coding systems were designed to classify or index medical information for research or other purposes, MEDCIN was designed for point-of-care usage by the clinician. MEDCIN is not just a list of medical terms, but rather a list of *findings* (clinical observations) that are medically meaningful to the clinician.

An EHR system based on MEDCIN enables the clinician to select fewer individual codes and to quickly locate other clinical "findings" that are likely to be needed. This difference reduces the time it takes to create exam notes and allows a physician to complete the patient exam note at the time of the encounter.

LOINC

LOINC stands for Logical Observation Identifiers Names and Codes. LOINC was created and is maintained by the Regenstrief Institute, which is closely affiliated with the Indiana University School of Medicine. LOINC standardizes codes for laboratory test orders and results, such as blood hemoglobin and serum potassium, and also clinical observations, such as vital signs or EKGs.

LOINC is important because currently most laboratories and other diagnostic services report test results using their own internal, proprietary codes. When an EHR receives results from multiple lab facilities, comparing the results electronically is like comparing apples and oranges. LOINC provides a universal coding system for mapping laboratory tests and results to a common terminology in the EHR. This then makes it possible for a computer program to find and report comparable test values regardless of where the test was processed.

Capturing and Recording EHR Data

The value of having an EHR is evident, but how does the data get into the EHR? Thus far we have discussed three forms of EHR data, digital images, text files, and discrete data. In subsequent chapters of this book we will explore how healthcare providers (clinicians, nurses, and medical assistants) create codified electronic health records. But before we move on, let us briefly examine how digital image data and text file data are added to the EHR and used. We will also discuss additional sources of EHR data that can be imported directly into the system.

Digital Image Systems

As discussed previously, digital image data can be subcategorized into diagnostic images and scanned document images. Even with the eventual total implementation of a codified EHR, EHRs will always have some paper documents. For example, the old paper charts of established patients need to be retained, and there will also be a continuing influx of referral letters and other paper medical documents from outside sources.

Many healthcare organizations choose to bring paper documents into the EHR as scanned images. Though scanned images do not offer all of the benefits of a codified medical record, they do provide widespread accessibility and a means to include source documents for a complete electronic chart.

Most document image systems have a computer program to associate various ID fields and keywords with scanned images. The process of associating these fields and keywords with images is called *cataloging the image*. Catalog data adds the ability to search an EHR for the electronic document images in multiple ways.

Guided Exercise 3: Exploring a Document Image System

In this exercise we are going to explore an imaging system. You will need access to the Internet for this exercise. If you have not already done so, complete the student registration for the MyHealthProfessionsKit provided on the inside cover of this book.

Step 1

Start your web browser program and follow the steps listed inside the cover of this textbook to select a discipline, click on the book cover that matches this Essentials of Electronic Health Records textbook, and login.

When the welcome page is displayed, click on the link "Activities and Exercises" or select "Activities" from the drop-down list and click on the button labeled "Go."

Step 2

A menu on the left of the screen will list various activities and exercises.

Locate and click on the link Exercise 3.

Information about the exercise will be displayed.

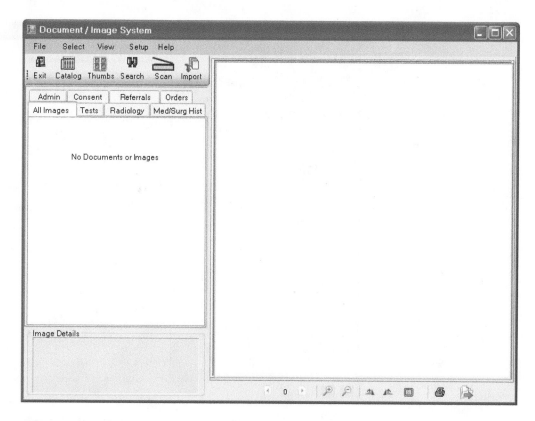

Locate and click the link "Click here to start the Document / Image System program." A screen similar to Figure 2-1 will be displayed.

The Document/Image System Window As you proceed through the following steps you will be introduced to names, functions and components of the Document/Image System window. This program simulates many of the features typically found in an EHR document image management system.

Menu Bar At the top of the screen, the words File, Select, View, Setup, and Help are the functions typically found in document image software. This is called the Menu bar. When you position the mouse over one of these words and click the mouse once, a list of functions will drop down below the word.

Once a menu list appears, clicking one of the items in the list will invoke that function. Clicking the mouse anywhere except on the list will close the list. Certain items on the menu are displayed in gray text. These items are not available until a patient or document has been selected. The Setup and Help options are not available in this simulation.

Step 3

Position the mouse pointer over the word Select in the Menu bar at the top of the screen and click the mouse button once. A list of the Select menu functions will appear (see Figure 2-2).

Step 4

Move the mouse pointer vertically down the list over the word "Patient" and click the mouse to invoke the Patient Selection window shown in Figure 2-3.

Step 5

Find the patient named Raj Patel in the Patient Selection window. Position the mouse pointer over the patient name and double-click the mouse. (Double-click means to click the mouse button twice, very rapidly.)

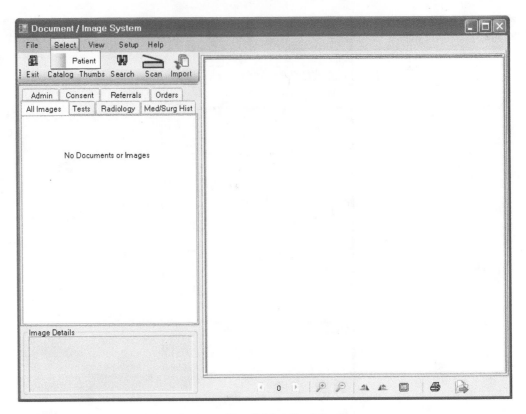

▶ Figure 2-2 **Document/Image System after clicking the Select menu.**

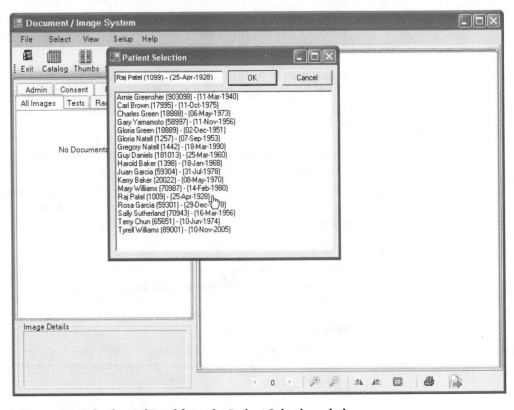

▶ Figure 2-3 **Selecting Raj Patel from the Patient Selection window.**

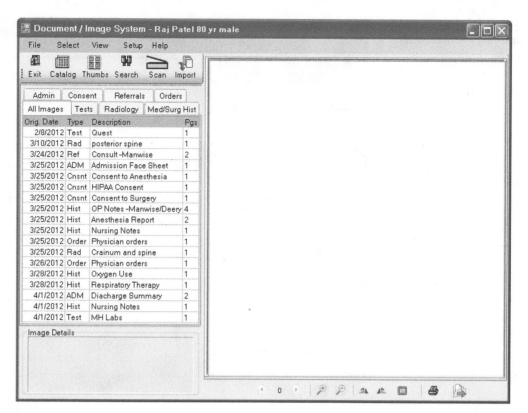

▶ Figure 2-4 **Left pane displays catalog list of documents and images for Raj Patel.**

Once a patient is selected, the patient's name, age, and sex are displayed in the Title bar at the top of the window.

Compare your screen to Figure 2-4 as you read the following information:

Toolbar Also located at the top of your screen are a row of icon buttons called a "Toolbar." The purpose of the Toolbar is to allow quick access to commonly used functions. Most Windows programs feature a Toolbar so you may already be familiar with the concept.

Catalog Pane The middle portion of the screen is divided into two window panes. The left pane (just below the Toolbar) is where a list of cataloged documents displays once a patient is selected. At the top of the catalog pane there are eight tabs. These look like tabs on file folders. The tabs are used to limit the list to images by category making it easier to find a specific type of image quickly. The initial tab is "All Images," listed in date order.

Step 6

Locate the Toolbar in the Document/Image System window. The first icon is labeled "Exit" and it will close the simulation program and return you to the MyHealthProfessionsKit page. Do not click it yet.

The next two buttons are used to change the display of items in the catalog pane from a list to thumbnails. Thumbnails are small versions of the document or image.

Position your mouse pointer over the "Thumbs" icon on the Toolbar (circled in Figure 2-5) and click your mouse.

! Alert

All instructions in these exercises refer to the simulation window. Because you are running this simulation inside a browser, be careful to use the Menu bar and Toolbar inside the simulation window, not the Menu bar or Toolbar of your Internet browser program.

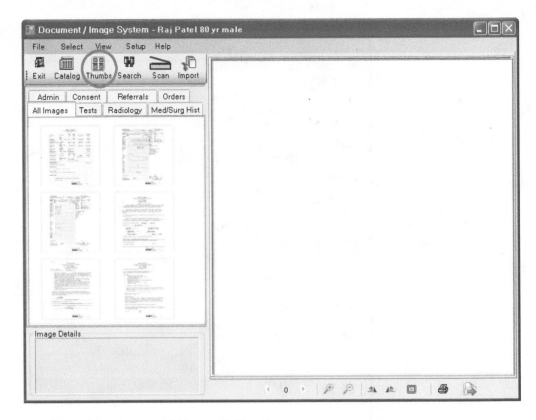

Compare your screen to Figure 2-5.

Now position your mouse pointer over the "Catalog" icon on the Toolbar and click your mouse. Your screen should again resemble Figure 2-4.

Step 7

Locate the tab labeled "Med/Srg Hist" above the Catalog pane. Position your mouse pointer over it and click your mouse. The list should now be shorter because it is limited to items cataloged in the category of Medical/Surgical History.

Step 8

Locate the catalog item "Anesthesia Report," and click on it. Compare your screen to Figure 2-6 as you read the following information:

Image Viewer Pane The right pane of the window will dynamically display the corresponding image for a catalog entry that is clicked.

Item Details Just below the Catalog pane is a gray panel that displays information about a selected catalog item such as the user who scanned the document, relevant dates, and a longer description of the item.

Image Tools Just below the Image Viewer pane is a row of icon buttons used to change the displayed image. These include the abilities to page through multipage documents and to enlarge or reduce the displayed image.

Step 9

Locate the image tools buttons just below the Image Viewer pane. The first three icons become active whenever a multipage document is selected. The anesthesia report has two pages. Locate and click on the Next page arrow button (circled in

► Figure 2-6 Catalog pane for the Med/Srg Tab at left; anesthesia report displayed in the Image Viewer pane at right.

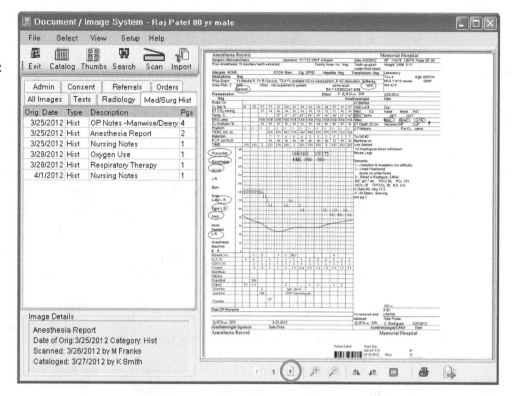

red in Figure 2-6). The button displays the next page of a multipage document. The numeral between the two arrow buttons is the page number currently displayed. Your screen should now display the second page of the report and the Image Tool should display the numeral "2."

The Previous page button is the first button in the image tools row. Locate it and click on it. The image tool area should now display the numeral "1," and the Image Viewer pane should again display the first page of the report.

The next two icons resemble magnifying glasses. One includes a plus sign, this is the Zoom In tool; it enlarges the text in the viewer. The other magnifying glass has a minus sign, this is the Zoom Out tool; it reduces the enlarged view to show more of the page in the viewer.

Locate and click on the Zoom In icon to see how this works.

Cataloging Images

The process of scanning documents or importing scanned images into an image system includes not only capturing the image, but tying it to the correct patient and entering data in the computer about the document such as the date, provider, type of image, and so on. This is called cataloging the image. Figure 2-10, shown later, is an example of an image catalog system.

Document images are scanned and cataloged into the EHR by many different people, including medical assistants and personnel in the patient registration and Health Information Management (HIM) departments. During scanning and cataloging, quality control is most important. Once a document has been scanned and cataloged, the original may be shipped to a remote storage facility or shredded. In either case the original document may no longer be available for comparison. Although the scanned document image is stored safely on the computer, if it has been incorrectly cataloged it may not be easy to locate.

Memorial Hospital
876 Memory Ln, Anywhere, ID 83776
(208) 378-5555
CONSENT TO USE AND DISCLOSE HEALTH INFORMATION
for Treatment, Payment, or Healthcare operations

I understand that as part of my healthcare, Memorial Hospital originates and maintains health records describing my health history, symptoms, examination and test results, diagnoses, treatment, and any plans for future care or treatment. I understand that this information serves as:

- a basis for planning my care and treatment
- a means of communication among the many health professionals who contribute to my care
- a source of information for applying my diagnosis and surgical information to my bill
- a means by which a third-party payer can verify that services billed were actually provided
- and a tool for routine healthcare operations such as assessing quality and reviewing the competence of healthcare professionals

I understand and have been provided with a *Notice of Privacy Practices* that provides a more complete description of information uses and disclosures. I understand that I have the right to review the notice prior to signing this consent. I understand that Memorial Hospital reserves the right to change their notice and practices and prior to implementation will mail a copy of any revised notice to the address I've provided. I understand that I have the right to object to the use of my health information for directory purposes. I understand that I have the right to request restrictions as to how my health information may be used or disclosed to carry out treatment, payment, or healthcare operations and that Memorial Hospital is not required to agree to the restrictions requested. I understand that I may revoke this consent in writing, except to the extent that the hospital and its employees have already take action in reliance thereon.

I request the following restrictions to the use or disclosure of my health information:

Signature of Patient or Legal Representative Witness

Date Notice Effective Date or Version

__X__ Accepted _____ Denied

Signature: ___Raj Patel___ Date: ___3-24-2011___

Patient: Patel, Raj
Med Rec #: 837155

► Figure 2-7 **HIPAA consent form with barcode at bottom.**

For the most part, catalog data are entered by hand, but in some instances the image cataloging can be automated. Here are some examples of automated image cataloging:

Paper forms can include a barcode to identify catalog data; the scanning software interprets the barcode and automatically creates the catalog record. For example, Figure 2-7 shows a HIPAA authorization form that was printed for a patient signature. The form includes a barcode identifying the patient, date, and document type, allowing automatic cataloging of the signed copy when it is scanned by the document image system.

Another type of technology uses optical character recognition (OCR) software to recognize text characters in images. Some document imaging systems can be programmed to find and use the text contained in the scanned document to populate the fields in the catalog records. Typically only a few types of documents are processed in this way because each document type requires custom programming. However, when an organization creates images of thousands of the same type of document, it can be worth it. For example, your bank keeps an image of the front and back of each check it processes. Because the account number and check number are in a consistent place at the bottom of the check, the bank's computers can automatically catalog each image to the correct account as it is scanned.

Guided Exercise 4: Importing and Cataloging Images

In this exercise you will catalog a scanned report and a diagnostic image for a patient. You will need access to the Internet for this exercise.

Step 1

If you are still logged in from the previous exercise, proceed to step 2, otherwise start your web browser program and follow the steps listed inside the cover of this textbook to select a discipline, click on the book cover that matches this Essentials of Electronic Health Records textbook, and login.

When the welcome page is displayed, click on the link "Activities and Exercises" or select "Activities" from the drop-down list and click on the button labeled "Go."

Locate and click on the link Exercise 4. Information about the exercise will be displayed.

Locate and click the link "Click here to start the Document / Image System program," as you did in the previous exercise.

The document image system screen will be displayed. (Refer to Figure 2-1 for an example.)

Step 2

Position your mouse pointer over the word Select in the Menu bar at the top of the screen and click the mouse button once.

Move the mouse pointer vertically down the list over the word "Patient" and click the mouse to invoke the Patient Selection window shown in Figure 2-8.

Step 3

Find the patient named Sally Sutherland in the Patient Selection window.

Position the mouse pointer over the patient name and double-click the mouse.

Once a patient is selected, the patient's name, age, and sex are displayed in the Title bar at the top of the window. The Catalog pane displays the message "No Documents or Images" because Sally has no documents or images in the catalog.

► Figure 2-8 Selecting Sally
Sutherland from the Patient
Selection window.

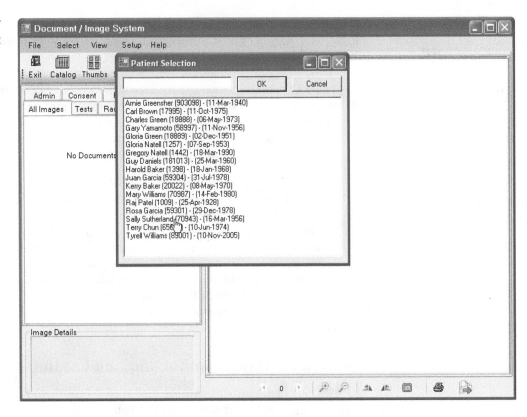

► Figure 2-8 **Selecting Sally
Sutherland from the Patient
Selection window.**

Step 4

Because you may not have a scanner connected to your computer, you are going
to import a file that has already been scanned, but not yet cataloged.

Locate and click on the Toolbar button labeled "Import." A window of available
files will open. Compare your screen to Figure 2-9.

► Figure 2-9 **Open Media
File window displays after
the clicking the Import icon.**

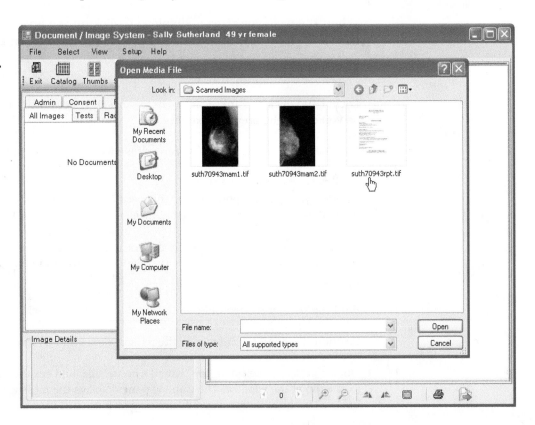

Step 5

Locate and click on the thumbnail image of the radiologist's report document ("suth70943rpt.tif").

Locate and click on the button labeled "Open." Compare your screen to Figure 2-10.

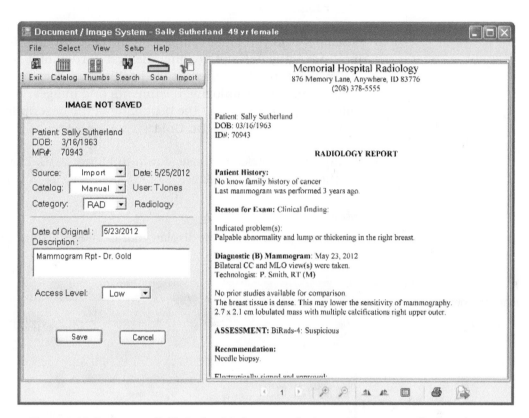

► Figure 2-10 **Data entry fields in the Catalog pane; the Image Viewer pane displays the imported radiology report.**

Step 6

The imported file displays in the Image Viewer pane and data entry fields replace the catalog list. The fields shown in Figure 2-10 are the minimum for most document imaging systems. The actual fields in a catalog record will differ by software vendor or medical facility.

The image you have imported should be the radiologist's report. The Catalog pane reminds you that it has not been saved into the patient's EHR.

The first two fields in the Catalog pane are determined automatically because the document imaging system recognizes that you have imported the file and that you are performing a manual entry of the catalog data. Other options for these fields are "Scanned" image and "Automatic" cataloging (e.g., from a barcode).

The Category field uses short mnemonic codes to represent longer category names, for example HIST for "Medical/Surgical History" or RAD for "Radiology." The Category field is already set to RAD.

The first field you will enter is the date of the original document. This is used for reference purposes to locate a document by the date of the report, letter, surgery, and so on. Note that the system will automatically record other dates, such as the date of the scan, the date it was cataloged, and so on. These other dates are used for audit purposes.

Look at the image displayed and locate the date of the report: May 23, 2012. Enter **5/23/2012**.

The final field you must complete is the description. Although, the field can hold a lengthy description, only the first portion of it is displayed in the catalog list, which is used by others at the healthcare facility to find the document/image. Therefore, when cataloging documents and images, be sure to put the most important information at the beginning of the description. In this case, you will type **Mammogram Rpt - Dr. Gold**.

Compare your fields to those shown in Figure 2-10. If everything is correct, click on the button labeled "Save."

Step 7

The Catalog pane will now display your cataloged listing (as shown in Figure 2-11).

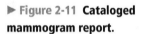 **Figure 2-11 Cataloged mammogram report.**

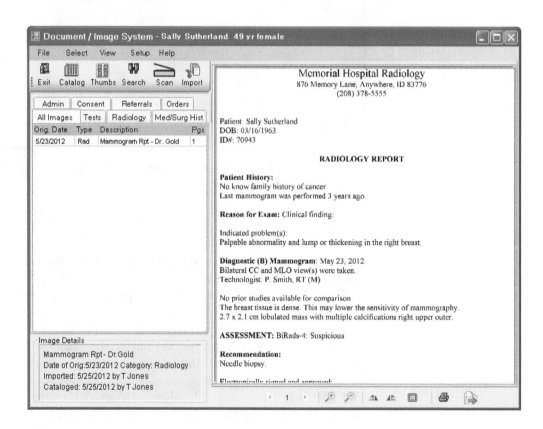

Now catalog the corresponding diagnostic images:

Locate and click on the Toolbar button labeled "Import." The Open Media File window (shown in Figure 2-9) will be displayed.

Click on the center thumbnail (the mammogram image "suth70943mam2.tif"). Locate and click on the button labeled "Open."

Enter the catalog data in the Catalog entry fields as follows:

Date: **5/23/2012**

Description: **Mammogram right breast w/abnormality**

Compare your left pane to Figure 2-12. Click the button labeled "Save."

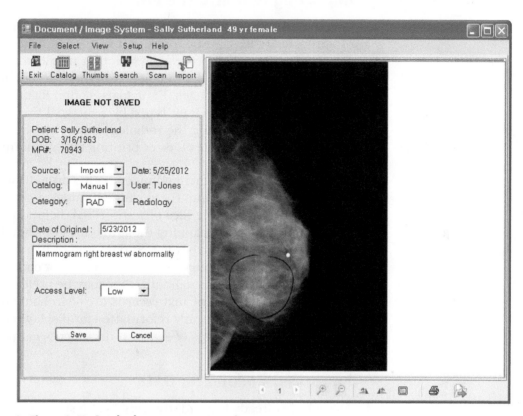

▶ Figure 2-12 **Cataloging a mammogram image.**

Step 8

Catalog another diagnostic image by again clicking the Toolbar button labeled "Import." When the Open Media File window appears, click on the leftmost thumbnail (the mammogram image "suth70943mam1.tif").

Locate and click on the button labeled "Open."

Enter the catalog data in the Catalog entry fields as follows:

Date: **5/23/2012**

Description: **Mammogram left breast**

Click the button labeled "Save." The Catalog pane will now display three listings.

The exercise is concluded. You may exit and close your browser.

Picture Archiving and Communication System

In the preceding exercise you imported diagnostic images (mammograms) into the EHR. At many facilities, digital images such as x-rays and CAT scans reside on a separate picture archiving and communication system (PAC.) These images can be associated with the radiology report in the EHR and appear to be part of the EHR record, even though they are on a separate system. In those facilities the diagnostic image is not actually imported into the EHR, but is instead linked to the patient EHR record.

Importing Text into the EHR

The second form of data we discussed is text data; that is, data that consists of words, sentences, and paragraphs, but is not fielded. Frequently this type of data comes from word processing files that result from transcribed dictation. A good example of this is the radiologist's report. A radiologist is a specialist who interprets diagnostic images. Radiologists often dictate their impressions of a study. Their dictation is later typed by a medical transcriptionist. The word processing file containing the radiology report can be imported directly into the EHR, eliminating the steps of printing and scanning.

Similarly, a healthcare facility implementing an EHR will eventually need to bring old paper charts into the document imaging system. If the facility has retained word processing files of transcribed dictation, importing them as EHR text records instead of scanning the printed pages from the paper chart increases the amount of the EHR that is text data and reduces the number of pages to be scanned. Although imported text data are not codified like those created when clinicians enter actual data, they may be preferable to a scanned image for two reasons. First, the text records are searchable by computer. Second, text data can be dynamically reformatted for display on smaller devices such as mobile phones; images of scanned documents cannot.

Importing Coded EHR Data

As we have already learned, the very best form of EHR data is codified, fielded data. In addition to the coded data that will be created by the clinician using an EHR, many other sources of codified data can be imported into the EHR system. Importing coded data produces a better EHR and eliminates the need to rekey data or scan reports into the chart.

For example, electronic lab order and results systems can be interfaced to send the orders and merge test results directly into the patient's chart. The numerical data that makes up many lab results lends itself to trend analysis, graphs, and comparison with other tests. The ability to review and present results in this manner allows providers to see the immediate, tangible benefits of using an EHR and also improves patient care.

Other sources of EHR data available for import into the EHR include vital signs when they are measured with modern electronic devices. Similarly glucose monitors and Holter monitors are devices that gather and store data about the patient. Most of these medical devices have the ability to transfer the data they have collected to the computer.

When clinicians use the EHR to write prescriptions, the orders are also automatically recorded in the EHR as part of the workflow. This keeps a record of the patient's past prescriptions and makes renewing prescriptions much faster for the provider.

Patient-Entered Data

Some medical practices use a program such as Instant Medical History™, developed by Dr. Allen Wenner, that allows patients to enter their history and symptom information on a computer in the waiting room or via the Internet prior to the visit. The patient-entered data is reviewed by the provider during the exam and then merged into the EHR.

Health Level 7

Health Level 7 (HL7) is a nonprofit organization and the leading messaging standard used by healthcare computer systems to exchange information. Hospitals and other large healthcare organizations often have many different computer systems that generate some portion of the patient medical data. HL7 is used to translate and interface that data into the main EHR system.

Regional Health Information Organization

One of the issues discussed in Chapter 1 was that patients often no longer see a single doctor, so their records reside in many separate specialists' offices. Efforts by RHIOs and by the Office of the National Coordinator for Health Information Technology to develop a national health information network are designed to allow for the electronic transfer of health records between providers.

Provider-Entered Data

Finally, the surest source of reliable coded EHR data is that entered by the providers (doctor, nurse, and medical assistant) during the patient encounter using a standardized nomenclature. That process will be the subject of Chapters 3 through 8 of this book.

Functional Benefits from Codified Records

Because coded EHR data is consistent in meaning, the computer can use it for trend analysis, alerts, health maintenance, decision support, orders and results, administrative processes, and population health reporting. We will now explore four of the functional benefits that can be derived from using a codified EHR.

Trend Analysis

In healthcare, laboratory tests are used to measure the level of certain components present in specimens taken from the patient. When the same test is performed over a period of time, changes in the results can indicate a *trend* in the patient's health.

With a paper chart, the clinician must page through the reports and mentally remember the values to compare them. When a health record is electronic, it is easier to compare data from different dates, tests, or events. When the data is fielded and coded, it is possible to generate graphs and reports that support trend analysis.

To experience the differences in forms of data we will compare a patient's lab results that have been stored in each of the three data formats we discussed earlier in this chapter.

Critical Thinking Exercise 5: Retrieving a Scanned Lab Report

In this exercise you will use what you have learned in Exercise 3 to locate information from a recent lab report for a patient.

Step 1

Start your web browser program and follow the steps listed inside the cover of this textbook to log in as you did in Exercise 3. Locate and select Exercise 5. Locate and click the link to start the Document / Image System program.

Step 2

Select patient "Raj Patel."

Step 3

On **February 8, 2012**, the facility received the results of a lab test performed by **Quest** laboratories. The lab report was scanned and cataloged in Raj Patel's chart.

Locate the catalog entry for this lab report and click on it to display the report.

Step 4

When the report is displayed in the Image Viewer pane, locate the results for the test component "Triglycerides" and write down the value on a sheet of paper with your name and today's date.

You may need to use the Zoom In button to read the value accurately.

Step 5

Close your browser window and give your paper to your instructor.

This is an example of data in the format of a digital image. As you can see the lab data are present in the EHR, but they require a human to locate and read the data values.

Lab Report as Text Data If a lab results report was received as a text file it might resemble Figure 2-13. The file could be imported into the EHR, but because the

```
Raj Patel                                              Page 1 of 1

Raj Patel: M: 3/6/1932:

Doctor's Laboratory
3/10/2012 11:30 AM

Tests
Blood Chemistry:                    Value              Normal Range
Total plasma cholesterol level      215 mg/dl          140 - 200
Plasma HDL cholesterol level        40 mg/dl           30 - 70
Plasma LDL cholesterol level        98 mg/dl           80 - 130
Total cholesterol/HDL ratio         5.4                4 - 6

Hematology:                         Value              Normal Range
INR                                 2.1                25 - 40
```

▶ Figure 2-13 **Lab results report in plain text.**

data in are not fielded or codified, a computer might have difficulty accurately parsing the data in the report. It could, however, easily search text records and locate those that contained the word "cholesterol." This could be useful to quickly locate records of previous tests containing the same word.

Coded Lab Data If the test result data is fielded and coded, the computer can find matching results in the data. One example of this is a cumulative summary report. These reports make it easier to compare test results from different times and dates.

The cumulative summary report shown in Figure 2-14 has three sections of results: blood gases, whole blood chemistries, and general chemistry. Within

```
*********************************************** Blood Gases ***********************************************

DATE:          [--------------------03/26/2012--------------------] 03/25/2012
TIME:          2132       1920       1720       1506       1615      NORMAL     UNITS

pH-Arterial    7.30 L     7.36       7.38       7.47 H     7.48 H    7.35-7.45
PCO2-Arterial  47.4 H     41.1       38.3       34.8 L     33.0 L    35-45      mm Hg
PO2-Arterial   90.2       189.0 H    187.0 H    188.0 H    227.0 H   90-105     mm Hg
HCO3-Arterial  22.8       22.8       22.0       24.9       24.4      21-27      mEq/L
Base Excess-A                                   1.7        1.6       0-3        mEq/L
Base Deficit-A 3.2 H      1.9        2.3                             0-3        mEq/L
O2 Sat Dir-A   96.0       99.3 H     99.5 H     99.6 H     99.9 H    95-99      % Saturation
O2 Content-A   15.9       15.3       14.6 L     10.3 L     14.4 L    15-17      vol %
Hemoglobin-BG  12.0       10.8       10.3       7.2        10.1                 g/dL
CarboxyHb-A    1.1 H      1.0 H      1.2 H      0.9        1.6 H     0.0-0.9    % Saturation
MetHb-A        0.9        0.4        0.7        0.4        0.8       0.0-0.9    % Saturation
FIO2                      .55        .56        0.54       .65                  %


*********************************** Whole Blood Chemistries ***********************************

DATE:          [--------------------- 03/26/2012 ---------------------] 03/25/2012
TIME:          2209     2132     1920     1720     1506     1615      NORMAL     UNITS

Sodium-WB                        142      142      142      139       135-145    mEq/L
Potassium-WB   3.5               3.3      3.0 L    2.9 L    2.7 L     3.3-4.6    mEq/L
Calcium Ionized         1.21     1.05     0.99 L   1.07     1.08      1.05-1.30  mmol/L
Lactic Acid-WB          1.3      0.8      1.1      0.8      0.5       0.3-1.5    mmol/L
Glucose-WB              197 H    156 H    165 H    118 H    90        65-99      mg/dL
Hematocrit-WB           37       34 L     32 L     22 L     31 L      36-46      %


*********************************** General Chemistry ***********************************

DATE:          04/01/2012 [---- 03/30/2012 ----] [--------- 03/29/2012 ---------]03/28/2012
TIME:          *0620    0653     0327     1835     0915     0532     2048     NORMAL     UNITS

Sodium         140                                         143               136-145    mmol/L
PotaSSium      2.7 L    3.0 L             2.9 L    3.0 L    2.7 L             3.3-5.1    mmol/L
Chloride       101                                         100               98-107     mmol/L
Carbon Dioxide 32 H                                        36 H              22-30      mmol/L
Urea Nitrogen  10                                          7                 6-20       mg/dL
Creatinine     0.54                                        0.60              0.40-0.90  mg/dL
Glucose        115 H                                       96                65-99      mg/dL
Calcium        8.4                                         8.0               8.0-10.6   mg/dL
Magnesium      1.9                                         2.3      1.8      1.5-2.8    mg/dL
Phosphorus Inorg 2.3 L                                     2.8      1.8 L    2.7-4.5    mg/dL
CK Total                         165                                273 H    30-170     U/L

-----------------------------------------------------------------------------------------
        H=Abnormal High          L=Abnormal Low          H*=Critical High          L*=Critical Low
        Date Printed: 04/01/2012          Admit Date: 03/25/2012          Discharge Date: 04/01/2012
                         INPATIENT MEDICAL RECORDS COPY                  Page: 1
```

▶ Figure 2-14 Cumulative summary lab report.

each section are the results from tests performed five different times; the date and time is printed above each column of data.

The report is read from left to right; each row contains the name of the test component followed by result values for each of the five times. The right two columns are informational; they contain the range of values considered normal for each particular test and the unit of measure.

It is only possible to generate meaningful cumulative summary reports when the data has uniform codes for tests and components.

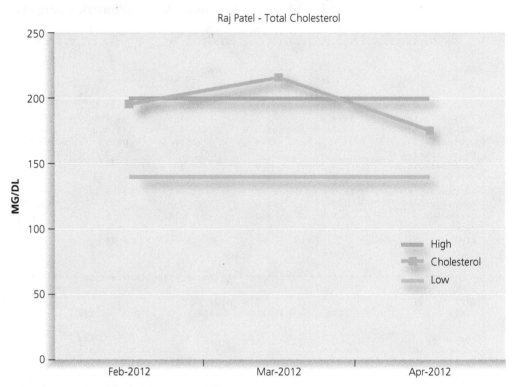

▶ Figure 2-15 **Graph of total cholesterol from codified lab results.**

A simple graphing tool can turn numeric data in the EHR into a powerful visual aid that would be impractical to create from a paper chart. Figure 2-15 provides an example of how data from multiple lab tests can be quickly extracted and graphed for the clinician. The value of the total cholesterol results over a three-month period of time is trended with the green line. The reference ranges of normal high (200) and low (140) values are shown in the graph as red and blue lines, respectively.

The computer is able to generate this graph because the data is fielded and the different tests and components have unique codes. From all of the possible tests a patient might have had, the computer can quickly find those coded as "total cholesterol." Using a graph, the clinician can easily see the trend in this patient's total cholesterol level.

Trend analysis is not limited to lab test results. Graphs of patient weight loss or gain are used as patient education tools. Effects of medication can be measured by comparing changes in dosage to changes in blood pressure measurements. Flow sheets are another type of trend analysis tool.

Alerts

One of the important reasons for the widespread adoption of EHRs is the potential to reduce medical errors. Paper charts and even electronic charts that are principally scanned images depend on the clinician noticing a risk factor about the patient. However, when an EHR consists primarily of fielded and codified data using standard nomenclature, rules can be set up that allow the computer to do the monitoring.

Alert is the term used in an EHR for a message or reminder that is automatically generated by the system. Alerts are based on programmed rules that cause the EHR to notify the provider when two or more conditions are met. For example, an electronic prescription system generates an alert when two drugs known to have adverse interactions are prescribed for the same patient.

Alert systems can be programmed for just about anything in the EHR. However, the most prevalent alert systems are those implemented with electronic prescription systems. Interactions between multiple prescription drugs, allergic reactions to certain classes of drugs, and patient health conditions that contraindicate certain drugs can all contribute to suffering, additional illness, and in extreme cases even death.

To prevent this, most physicians consult the patient medication list, allergy list, and the *Physicians' Desk Reference* (for interactions) before writing a prescription. As a further precaution, the pharmacy checks for drug conflicts and provides the patient with warning materials about the drug. When prescriptions are written electronically, however, the computer can quickly and efficiently check for drug safety and present the clinician with warnings, alerts, and explanatory information about the risks of particular drugs. Figure 2-16 shows a clinical warning alert generated by the Allscripts EHR system. Let's take a closer look at how this process works.

▶ Figure 2-16 **Electronic prescription DUR alert.**

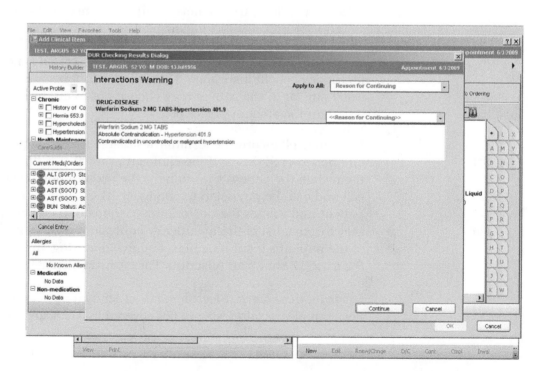

Drug Utilization Review When the clinician writing an electronic prescription selects a drug and enters the Sig[1] information, the EHR system scans the patient chart for allergy information, past and current diagnoses, and a list of current medications. This information is then passed to a drug utilization review (DUR) program that compares the prescription to a database of most known drugs. The database includes prescription drugs as well as over-the-counter drugs, and even nutritional herb and vitamin supplements. The DUR program performs the following functions:

♦ The drug about to be prescribed is checked against the patient medication list to determine if there is a conflict with any drug the patient is already taking. Certain drugs remain in the body for a period of time after the patient has stopped taking it. This latency period is factored in as well.

♦ Ingredients that make up the drug are checked against the ingredients of current medications to see if they conflict or would hinder the effectiveness of the drug.

♦ Drugs are checked for duplicate therapy, which occurs when a patient is taking a different drug of the same class that would have the effect of an overdose.

♦ Allergy records are checked for food and drug allergies that would be aggravated by the new drug.

♦ Some drugs cannot be given to patients with certain medical conditions; the patient's diagnosis history is checked to see if such a situation would occur.

♦ A patient education alert is created when the drug might be affected by certain foods or alcohol interactions.

♦ If the Sig has been entered at the time of the DUR, then it is also checked to see if it matches recommended guidelines for the drug. Too much, too little, too many days, or too many refills could cause overdosing, underdosing (causing it to be ineffective), or abuse.

If the DUR software finds any of these conditions, the clinician is given an alert message explaining the conflict. The clinician can then alter the prescription or select a new drug, having never issued the incorrect one.

Formulary Alerts Another type of alert found in many EHR prescription systems warns the clinician if the drug about to be prescribed is not covered by a patient's pharmacy benefit insurance. This is important because if a patient's insurance won't pay for it, the patient may choose not to fill the prescription or to take less than the amount prescribed.

Insurance plans provide formularies (lists) indicating preferred, nonpreferred, and noncovered drugs. If the clinician prescribes a drug that is not on the list, then when the patient tries to have the prescription filled, the pharmacy will call and ask the physician to change it. This causes an inconvenience to the patient and wastes the doctor's time. Instead, a clinician using an EHR can select from a list of therapeutically equivalent drugs that are on the formulary of the patient's insurance plan and avoid writing an incorrect prescription. Figure 2-17 shows an Allscripts Therapeutic Alternatives alert.

Other Types of Alerts Electronic lab order systems can provide alerts as well. For example, certain tests are not covered by Medicare. The Centers for Medicare

---

[1]The term *Sig*, from the Latin *signa*, refers to the instructions for labeling a prescription.

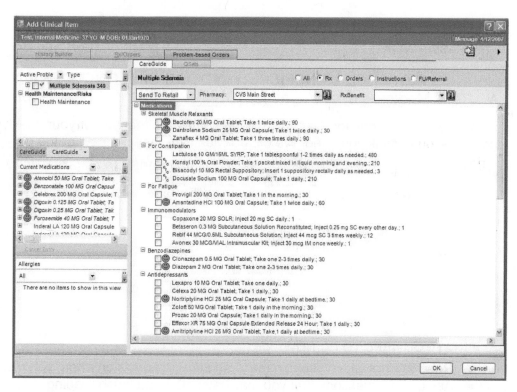

Courtesy of Allscripts, LLC

▶ Figure 2-17 **Electronic prescription formulary alert.**

and Medicaid Services (CMS), which is part of the U.S. Department of Health and Human Services (HHS), requires that patients sign a waiver indicating that they were notified that a test would not be covered. The waiver is called an Advance Beneficiary Notice (ABN). The sample form is shown in Figure 2-18. When certain tests are ordered, the clinician is alerted if an ABN is required.

Another example is an alert that monitors changes in values of certain blood tests and pages a doctor whenever the value is outside of a certain range.

Alerts can be generated by nonactions as well. Task list systems can notify an administrator when medical items are not handled in a timely fashion. Computerized provider order entry (CPOE) systems can generate alerts when results for a pending test order have not been received within the time frame normally required for that type of test.

Once an EHR system contains codified data, an alert system is just a matter of programming a rule to watch for a certain event or detect a finding with a value above or below the desired limit.

Health Maintenance

One of the best ways to maintain good health is to prevent disease, or if it occurs, to detect it early enough to be easily treated. Two important components of health maintenance are preventive care screening and immunizations.

Preventive Care The simplest example of health maintenance is a card or letter reminding the patient that it is time for a checkup. In a paper-based office, creating this reminder is a manual process. However, when a medical practice has electronic records, preventive screening can become more dynamic and sophisticated.

(A) Notifier(s):
(B) Patient Name: **(C) Identification Number:**

ADVANCE BENEFICIARY NOTICE OF NONCOVERAGE (ABN)

<u>NOTE</u>: If Medicare doesn't pay for **(D)**_____ below, you may have to pay.

Medicare does not pay for everything, even some care that you or your health care provider have good reason to think you need. We expect Medicare may not pay for the **(D)**_____ below.

(D)_____	**(E) Reason Medicare May Not Pay:**	**(F) Estimated Cost:**

WHAT YOU NEED TO DO NOW:

- Read this notice, so you can make an informed decision about your care.
- Ask us any questions that you may have after you finish reading.
- Choose an option below about whether to receive the **(D)**_____ listed above.
  Note: If you choose Option 1 or 2, we may help you to use any other insurance that you might have, but Medicare cannot require us to do this.

(G) OPTIONS: **Check only one box. We cannot choose a box for you.**

❑ **OPTION 1.** I want the **(D)**_____ listed above. You may ask to be paid now, but I also want Medicare billed for an official decision on payment, which is sent to me on a Medicare Summary Notice (MSN). I understand that if Medicare doesn't pay, I am responsible for payment, but **I can appeal to Medicare** by following the directions on the MSN. If Medicare does pay, you will refund any payments I made to you, less co-pays or deductibles.

❑ **OPTION 2.** I want the **(D)**_____ listed above, but do not bill Medicare. You may ask to be paid now as I am responsible for payment. **I cannot appeal if Medicare is not billed**.

❑ **OPTION 3.** I don't want the **(D)**_____ listed above. I understand with this choice I am **not** responsible for payment, and **I cannot appeal to see if Medicare would pay.**

(H) Additional Information:

This notice gives our opinion, not an official Medicare decision. If you have other questions on this notice or Medicare billing, call **1-800-MEDICARE** (1-800-633-4227/**TTY**: 1-877-486-2048).

Signing below means that you have received and understand this notice. You also receive a copy.

(I) Signature:	**(J) Date:**

According to the Paperwork Reduction Act of 1995, no persons are required to respond to a collection of information unless it displays a valid OMB control number. The valid OMB control number for this information collection is 0938-0566. The time required to complete this information collection is estimated to average 7 minutes per response, including the time to review instructions, search existing data resources, gather the data needed, and complete and review the information collection. If you have comments concerning the accuracy of the time estimate or suggestions for improving this form, please write to: CMS, 7500 Security Boulevard, Attn: PRA Reports Clearance Officer, Baltimore, Maryland 21244-1850.

Form CMS-R-131 (03/08)   Form Approved OMB No. 0938-0566

▶ Figure 2-18 **Sample Advance Beneficiary Notice form.**

Health maintenance systems, also known as preventive care systems, can go beyond simple reminders for an annual checkup. When an EHR has codified data, it can be electronically compared to the recommendations of the U.S. Preventive Services Task Force.

The U.S. Preventive Services Task Force is an independent panel of experts in primary care and prevention that systematically reviews the evidence of effectiveness and develops recommendations for clinical preventive services.

The task force makes recommendations about preventive services based on age, sex, and risk factors for disease. Research has shown that the best way to ensure that preventive services are delivered appropriately is to make evidence-based information readily available at the point of care. The task force recommendations have been incorporated in EHR systems from several vendors.

Using a sophisticated set of rules, the EHR software compares the list of tests recommended for patients of a certain age and sex to previous test results stored in the EHR. It also calculates the time since the test was last performed and compares that to the recommended interval for repeat testing. A guideline unique to the patient is generated and displayed on the clinician's computer. Using this information, the clinician can order tests, discuss important healthcare options, and recommend lifestyle changes to the patient at the point of care. Figure 2-19 shows the Health Maintenance screen from EHR vendor NextGen.

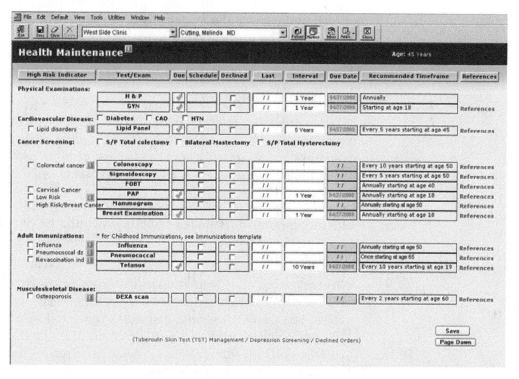

Courtesy of NextGen Healthcare

▶ Figure 2-19 **Health Maintenance screen.**

It would be difficult to create standardized rules for a preventive care system if the tests were not coded using a standardized coding system. Preventive care screening guidelines are not limited to lab tests; other examples include mammograms, hearing and vision screening, and certain elements of the physical examination.

Immunizations The other important component of preventive care is immunizations. Immunization slows down or stops disease outbreaks by vaccinating the population. Vaccination prevents disease in the people who receive the vaccine and protects those who come into contact with unvaccinated individuals.

Immunizations must be acquired over time. Vaccines cannot be given all at once. Several require repeated applications over a period of time, and some such as the measles vaccine cannot be given to children under the age of 1 year. Therefore, the Centers for Disease Control and Prevention (CDC) and state health departments have designed a schedule to immunize children and adolescents from birth through 18 years of age. The CDC also publishes a recommended immunization schedule for adults. Adult immunizations are different from those given to a child.

Using the codified data in an EHR, computers can compare a patient's immunization history with the CDC list of vaccines and recommended intervals to identify which immunizations the patient needs. EHR systems can also scan the data and generate letters to send to patients who have not been in recently but may need to renew their immunizations.

Decision Support

Physicians are trained to analyze information from a patient's history, physical exams, and test results for a medical decision. They are also accustomed to researching the medical literature when faced with an unusual case. However, the quantity of information available to clinicians regarding conditions, disease management, protocols, case studies, and treatments far exceeds their available time to read it.

Decision support refers to the ability of EHR systems to store or quickly locate materials relevant to the findings of the current case. These might include defined protocols, results of case studies, or standard care guidelines prepared by specialists, medical societies, or government organizations.

Decision support is not about "artificial intelligence" replacing a physician with a computer; it is instead about providing help just when the clinician needs it. There are many examples of decision support systems, but let us look at four:

◆ **Prescriptions:** Decision support can include the drug formularies mentioned earlier. Formularies can be used to look up drugs by name or therapeutic class. Electronic prescription systems provide decision support to the clinician by comparing alternative brands that are therapeutically equivalent. They can also provide information on costs, indications for use, treatment recommendations, dosage, guidelines, and prescribing information.

◆ **Medical References:** Decision support systems can provide quick access to medical references directly from the EHR. This can make access to evidence-based guidelines or medical literature as easy as clicking on a link in the chart.

◆ **Protocols:** Protocols are one form of decision support that can ultimately speed up documentation of the patient exam and improve patient care.

Protocols are standard plans of therapy established for different conditions. With a decision support system, when a doctor has diagnosed a patient with a particular condition, the appropriate protocol appears on the EHR screen and all therapies can be ordered with a click of the mouse.

◆ **Medication Dosing:** Many medications have serious side effects, some of which must be monitored by regular blood tests. When both the medications and lab results are stored in the EHR as codified data, it is possible for decision support software to compare changes in medication dosing with changes in the patient's test results. This assists the clinician in adjusting the patient's medication levels to obtain the maximum benefit to the patient.

Meeting the IOM Definition of an EHR

Each of the functional benefits we have discussed—trend analysis, alerts, health maintenance, and decision support—are products of EHR systems that store medical records as codified, fielded data. It is only when these functional benefits are added to the clinical practice that the EHR approaches the vision of the IOM discussed in Chapter 1.

Chapter Two Summary

The IOM definition of an EHR went beyond a computer file that just stores a patient's medical record to include the *functional benefits* derived from having an electronic health record. In this chapter we explored how the format in which the data are stored determines to what extent the data can be used to achieve that extended functionality.

The forms of EHR data are broadly categorized into three types:

1. Digital image data (provides increased accessibility)

2. Text-based data (provides accessibility, text search capability, and can be displayed on different devices)

3. Discrete data, fielded and ideally codified (provides all of the above plus the capability to be used for alerts, health maintenance, and data exchange). The increased benefits of an EHR can be realized when the information is stored as codified data. In addition, codified EHR data that adheres to a national standard enables the exchange and comparison of medical information from other facilities.

When EHR data is coded, it can be used for:

◆ **Trend analysis**—the comparison of multiple values or findings over a period of time

◆ **Alerts**—computer-prompted warnings such as a potential drug interaction or a lab result seriously above or below the expected range

◆ **Health maintenance**—computer-generated reminders of health screenings, immunizations, and other preventive measures.

◆ **Decision support**—systems that quickly locate materials relevant to the findings of the current case such as defined protocols, standard care guidelines, or medical research.

Testing Your Knowledge of Chapter 2

1. What is the advantage of codified data over document imaged data?

2. What does the acronym SNOMED-CT stand for?

3. What university is closely affiliated with the development of LOINC?

Give examples for the following terms:

4. Trend analysis

5. Decision support

6. Alerts

7. Health maintenance

8. List at least two ways codified data in the EHR can be used to manage and prevent disease.

9. What is a nomenclature?

10. What does the phrase *cataloging an image* refer to?

11. What does the acronym DUR stand for?

12. Name at least four things that a DUR checks.

13. What is an RHIO?

14. Name a type of alert other than prescription or drug alerts.

15. Name a type of decision support.

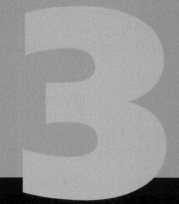

Learning Medical Record Software

Learning Outcomes

After completing this chapter, you should be able to:

◆ Start and stop the Student Edition software

◆ Navigate the screen

◆ Select a patient

◆ Create a new encounter

◆ Access the Symptoms, History, Physical Exam, Assessment, and Therapy tabs to add appropriate findings in each portion of a SOAP note

◆ Select findings and edit findings

◆ Remove findings

◆ Add entry details, values, free text, results, status, and episodes to findings

◆ Enter a chief complaint

◆ Enter vital signs

Introducing the Student Edition Software

In this chapter you will learn to document a patient encounter using Medcin, one of the standard EHR nomenclatures discussed in Chapter 2. Special Student Edition software has been created for you to use with this course. It is similar to many commercial software packages that use the Medcin knowledgebase for their EHR nomenclature.

The Student Edition software allows you select findings for symptoms, history, physical examination, tests, diagnoses, and therapy to produce medical documents typical of the clinical notes created in a medical office. At the conclusion of certain exercises, you will print out your work and give it to your instructor.

Because the Student Edition is not a commercial medical record system, it will be different in some aspects from the EHR systems you will use when working in a medical office specialty clinic or hospital setting. However, the concepts, skills, and familiarity with EHR systems you will acquire by practicing with the Student Edition software will transfer directly to the workplace.

One goal of most EHR systems is to completely document the encounter at the point of care delivery in a clinic or hospital or before the patient ever leaves the office in an outpatient setting. Once you have mastered the basics, you will learn in subsequent chapters how to increase your data entry speed through the use of lists and forms. These capabilities are useful for quickly documenting a patient visit during the encounter.

About the Exercises in This Book

The purpose of the exercises is to teach EHR concepts by providing hands-on experience. Completing the exercises in this and subsequent chapters of the book using the software provided will give you practical experience in creating electronic health records. Each set of exercises is designed to illustrate an EHR concept and will result in a documented clinical note.

Note, however, that many of the exercises cover portions of the visit that are not typically entered by a medical assistant, such as orders, assessment, and plan of treatment. The reason for including these components in the exercises is to help you understand the complete SOAP note. Note, too, that although the clinical notes produced by the exercises are medically accurate, they do not necessarily represent a thorough medical exam. Exercises may omit certain routine elements of the exam that would normally be documented. This is not a limitation of the Medcin knowledge base or of the physicians who reviewed the exercises. This is done solely to facilitate completion of exercises in the allotted class time.

Understanding the Software

The following series of exercises are designed to allow you to become familiar with the Student Edition software, the Medcin nomenclature, and the screen navigation controls. Do not worry if you cannot complete all of them in one class period.

Guided Exercise 6: Starting Up the Software

The Student Edition software should have been installed on your school's network computers or on your local workstation. If you are working on your own computer, and have not already installed the Student Edition software, follow the software download instructions inside the front cover before proceeding.

Step 1

Turn on the computer and wait for the Windows operating system desktop to appear on the screen. If you are using a school computer, you may be required to log in; if so, ask your instructor for the correct log-in procedure.

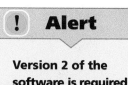

▶ Figure 3-1 **The Medcin Student Edition icon.**

Step 2

Locate the Medcin icon shown in Figure 3-1. If you do not see it on the computer desktop screen, click on the Start button, and look in Programs or All Programs for the program named "Medcin Student Edition."

Position the mouse pointer over the Medcin icon shown in Figure 3-1 and double-click the mouse button. This will display the Student Edition log-in screen shown in Figure 3-2.

▶ Figure 3-2 **Student Edition log-in screen.**

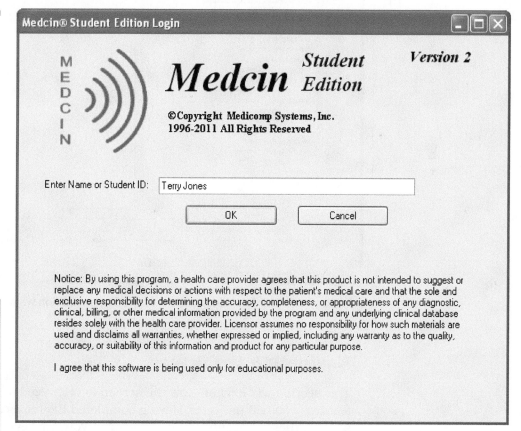

> ! **Alert**
>
> **Version 2 of the software is required for this text. If Version 2 is not displayed in the upper right corner of the log-in screen, stop and inform your instructor at once.**

Step 3

Figure 3-2 shows the Medcin Student Edition log-in screen. The screen contains one data entry field and two buttons. The field is used for either the student's name or the student ID depending on the policy of the school. In the example, the student's name is Terry Jones. Do not type Terry Jones in the field; confirm with your instructor whether you should use your name or student ID.

Type either your name or student ID into the field.

When your name or ID is exactly as you want it to be, position the mouse pointer over the button labeled "OK," and click the mouse button.

The button labeled "Cancel" is used to cancel the log in and close the window.

The main window of the Student Edition software will be displayed, as shown in Figure 3-3.

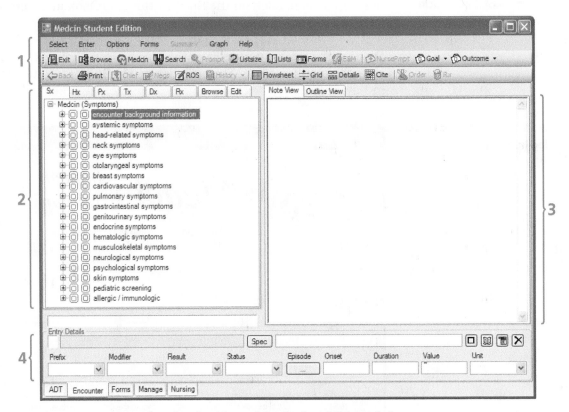

▶ Figure 3-3 **Four functional sections of the Student Edition window.**

Navigating the Screen

This section will explain how the screen is organized and discuss some of the features you will use later. Having completed Exercises 3, 4, and 5 in Chapter 2, some of these concepts will be familiar to you. However the Document/Image System simulation is not the same software as the Student Edition software program. It is only similar in appearance.

The main window can be divided into four functional sections. These four sections interact with each other as you will learn in this chapter. Refer to Figure 3-3 and locate each of the sections indicated by the red numerals 1 through 4.

Section 1: Menu Bar and Toolbar At the top of the screen, the words Select, Enter, Options, Forms, Summary, Graph, and Help are the menus of functions in the Student Edition software. As you learned in the previous chapter, when you position the mouse pointer over one of these words and click the mouse once, a list of functions will drop down below the word. Once a list appears, moving the mouse pointer vertically over the list will highlight each item. In the Student Edition, *highlight* refers to the colored rectangle that appears over an item. Clicking on the highlighted item will invoke that function. Clicking the mouse anywhere on the screen other than the list will close the list.

Also located at the top of your screen are two rows of icon buttons called a "Toolbar." The purpose of the Toolbar is to allow quick access to commonly used functions. Toolbar buttons will be identified later in the chapter, as you learn to use them.

Section 2: Medcin Nomenclature Pane The middle portion of the screen is divided into two window panes. The left pane (shown in Figure 3-3 with the numeral 2) displays findings in the Medcin nomenclature. In the next exercise, you will select a patient and learn to navigate the Medcin nomenclature pane.

At the top of the nomenclature pane there are eight tabs. These look like tabs on file folders. The first six of these are labeled: Sx (symptoms), Hx (history), Px (physical examination), Tx (tests), Dx (diagnosis, syndromes, and conditions), and Rx (therapy). The tabs are used to logically group the findings into six broad categories. Two additional tabs labeled Browse and Edit will be explained later as you use it the software.

Section 3: The Encounter View Pane The right pane of the window (shown in Figure 3-3 with the numeral 3) will dynamically display the patient encounter note as it is being created. When a healthcare professional selects a finding from the nomenclature pane, the finding and relevant accompanying text are recorded in the encounter note, which is displayed in the pane on the right.

Free text also may be entered through the software, and it will appear in the note view pane as well. This will become clearer during subsequent exercises. Because you have not yet selected a patient or an encounter, the pane is empty at this time.

There are two tabs on the top of the right pane. The Note View tab displays the encounter note in SOAP format as you create it. The Outline View tab displays findings that have been selected as well as appropriate ICD-9-CM or CPT-4 codes.

Section 4: Entry Details for a Current Finding The bottom portion of the screen (shown in Figure 3-3 with the numeral 4) consists of two rows of fields that allow the user to add detail to any finding recorded in the right pane. Entry of data in these fields adds informational text to the finding in the encounter note, and in some cases modifies its meaning.

For example, a patient-reported symptom of "headaches" could be modified using the Entry Details field labeled "Status" to indicate the condition was "improving." The meaning of the finding could be altered completely by use of the Entry Details field labeled "Prefix" to indicate "family history of." This would indicate that the patient did not have this condition, but that it had been a problem for close relatives. Each of the fields in the Entry Details section of the screen will be covered in subsequent exercises in this book.

To actually see the interactions of the four sections of the screen, you need to select a patient and create a new encounter. Subsequent exercises will show you how to do that, but first let us discuss exiting the software.

Guided Exercise 7: Exiting and Restarting the Software

There are three ways to exit the Student Edition software. In this exercise, you will practice exiting the software. You will then restart the program to continue with subsequent exercises.

At the top of your screen is a row of words called the Menu bar. Below it are two rows of buttons with icons, called the Toolbar. The first button in the Toolbar is labeled "Exit"; its icon looks like an open door. If you click on the Exit button, the Student Edition program will end and the window will close.

In the upper right corner of the window are three buttons that are standard to all Windows programs. From left to right, these buttons minimize, maximize, and close the window. The Close button is red, with a large X. If you click on the Close button, the Student Edition program will end and the window will close.

A third way to close the program is explained next.

Step 1

The first word in the Menu bar is "Select." Position the mouse pointer over the word Select in the Menu bar at the top of the screen and click the mouse button once. A list of the functions on the Select menu will drop down.

You will notice some of the items in the menu are listed in black text and some of them are in gray text. Menu items in gray text indicate that a particular function is not applicable to the current state of the encounter note and is therefore not selectable. You may have noticed some of the buttons on the Toolbar also are gray; this is for the same reason.

Step 2

Move the mouse pointer vertically down the list until the Exit function is highlighted. Click the mouse on the word "Exit" to end the program.

Step 3

Start the Student Edition software again by repeating Exercise 6 and logging in.

Guided Exercise 8: Using the Menu to Select a Patient

Once you are logged in, the first step in every encounter is to select the patient.

Step 1

Position the mouse pointer over the word Select in the Menu bar at the top of the screen and click the mouse button once. A list of the Select menu functions will appear (see Figure 3-4).

Step 2

Move the mouse pointer vertically down the list until Patient is highlighted. Click the mouse on the word Patient to invoke the Patient Selection window shown in Figure 3-5.

Step 3

The student edition Patient Selection window displays a list of all patients in the system, their last name, first name, patient ID number, and date of birth. A field at the top of the window allows you to type the patient's last name to quickly find someone in a large list.

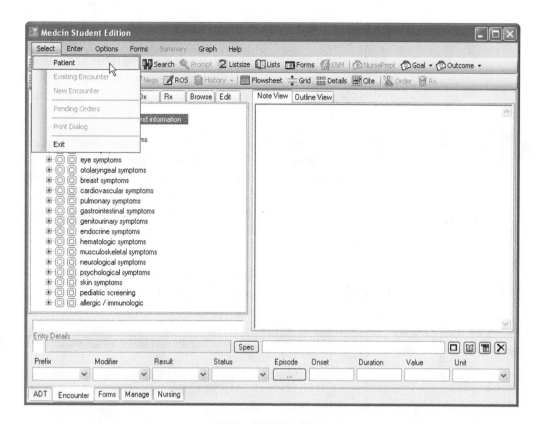

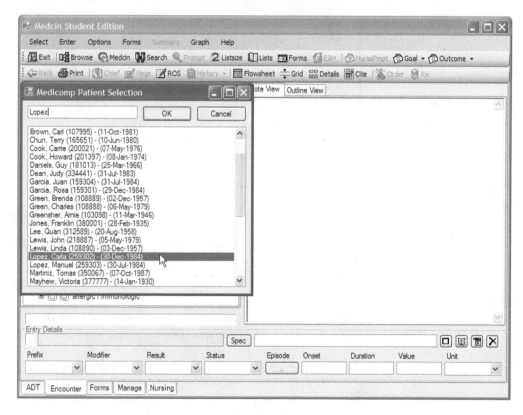

Find the patient named Carla Lopez in the Patient Selection window by typing **Lopez** in the field. When you start typing the name, the first name beginning with an "L" will be highlighted. As you continue to type, the next alphabetical name will be highlighted. When Carla Lopez is highlighted, click the OK button.

Clicking the Cancel button will close the window.

An alternate method of selecting the patient is to visually locate the patient's name, position the mouse pointer over it and double-click the mouse. (Double-click means to click the mouse button twice, very rapidly.)

Step 4

Once a patient is selected, the patient's name is displayed in the title at the top of the window (see Figure 3-6).

▶ Figure 3-6 **Left pane displays Medcin nomenclature.**

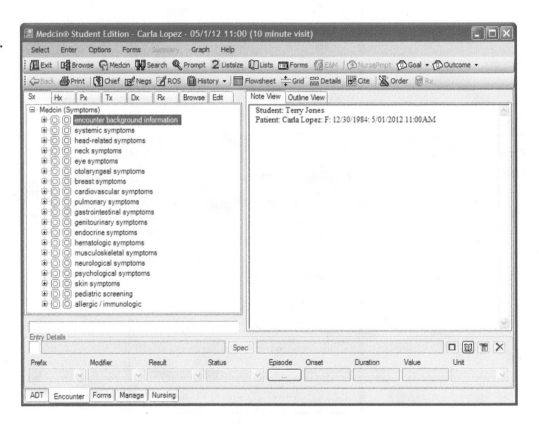

The right pane containing the encounter note is populated with the student's name or ID and the patient's name, sex, and date of birth.

Guided Exercise 9: Navigating the Medcin Findings

In this exercise, you will have an opportunity to become familiar with one way to navigate the Medcin nomenclature. In a subsequent exercise, you will learn to record the findings from the left pane into the encounter note in the right pane. In this exercise, you will not yet record any findings.

Your screen should resemble Figure 3-6. If it does not, repeat Exercise 8.

Step 1

Look at the list of findings in the left pane. As mentioned earlier, the pane on the left of the screen is used to select findings to document the current patient encounter.

The Medcin nomenclature consists of more than 277,000 findings with an estimated 68 million relationships. To make it easy to find what you are looking for, the tabs on the top of the left pane categorize findings into six broad groups that follow the order of a typical medical examination.

Chapter 1 described the SOAP format standard for documenting medical records. The six tabs at the top of the left pane make it easy to document in that format as follows:

Subjective	Sx	Symptoms
	Hx	History
Objective	Px	Physical exam
	Tx	Tests (performed)
Assessment	Dx	Diagnosis
Plan	Rx	Therapy, plan, and tests (ordered)

In addition to the tabs, another feature that shortens the list of findings displayed in the nomenclature pane is to show only the main topics.

You will notice that most findings in the Medcin list are preceded by buttons. These are shown in Figure 3-7. The symbols on the buttons are a small plus sign, a larger button with a red circle, and a larger button with blue circle.

The small plus sign indicates that more specific findings that are related to the finding that is displayed are hidden from view.

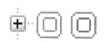

▶ Figure 3-7 **Buttons used in the Nomenclature pane.**

Step 2

Locate the finding "head-related symptoms" in the nomenclature symptoms list, as shown in Figure 3-8. Position the mouse pointer over the small plus symbol and click the mouse button once.

Compare the left pane of your screen with Figure 3-9. The list should have expanded to reveal many additional head-related findings. Notice that the findings under "head-related symptoms" are indented.

Notice also that some of the additional findings have small plus symbols as well, for example, "headache" and "pain behind the ear." This indicates that even more specific findings are available for those items. Conversely, findings such as "skull pain" and "scalp swelling" do not have the small plus sign. This means that no additional specific findings are available for those items.

Step 3

Position the mouse pointer over the small plus symbol for the finding "headache" in the indented list, and click the mouse. The list expands further.

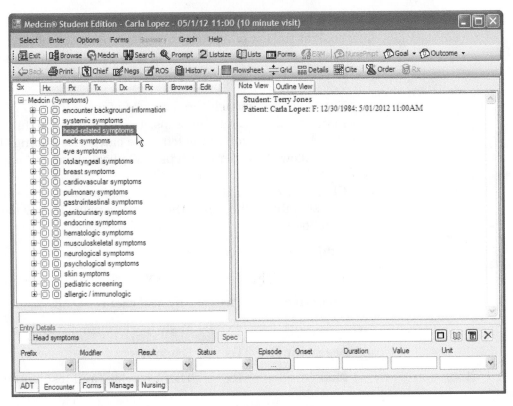

► Figure 3-8 **Locate the finding "head-related symptoms."**

► Figure 3-9 **Expanded list of findings for "head-related symptoms."**

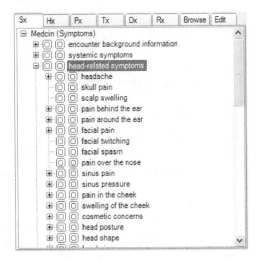

Step 4

Notice that many of these detailed findings, such as "location," "quality," "severity," "duration," and "timing," still have small plus symbols indicating that even further detailed findings are available.

Position the mouse pointer over the small plus symbol for the finding "timing" and click the mouse.

Position the mouse pointer over the small plus symbol for the finding "chronic/recurring" and click the mouse. Compare your list to Figure 3-10.

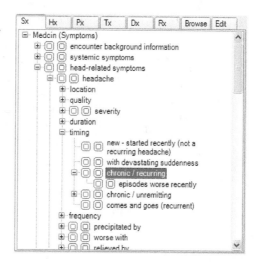

This type of list is called a *tree* because each indention of the list represents smaller branches of the finding above it. Look again at Figure 3-10; notice how each new level is indented further than the one above it. You may already be familiar with this concept because it is used in many other computer programs, including the Windows® operating system.

Each time you clicked on the small plus symbol next to a finding in steps 2, 3, and 4 the list grew. The term we use for this is that the tree has *expanded*. Also notice that a small minus sign replaced the small plus sign in the button next to any finding that has been expanded.

Step 5

Position the mouse pointer over the small minus symbol next to the finding "head-related symptoms" and click the mouse button again. The expanded list of various types of head-related symptom findings will again be hidden from view. Your screen should once again look like Figure 3-8.

When you clicked on the small minus symbol for the main finding, the number of findings for "head-related symptoms" was reduced back to one. The term we use for this is that the view of the tree has been *collapsed*. *Expand* and *collapse* are the terms that will be used in the exercises throughout this book when guiding your navigation of the Nomenclature pane.

Guided Exercise 10: Tabs on the Medcin Nomenclature Pane

Step 1

Position the mouse pointer over the Hx tab (circled in red in Figure 3-11) and click the mouse once.

The list will change to that shown in Figure 3-11. Notice that the currently selected tab has the appearance of being slightly raised from the others.

Step 2

Position the mouse pointer over the small plus next to "past medical history" and click the mouse button to expand the list.

► Figure 3-11 **The History tab.**

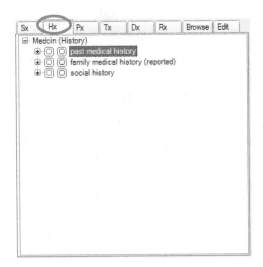

Step 3

Position the mouse pointer over the small plus next to "reported medications" and click the mouse button to expand the list. Notice that this time there were too many findings to fit in the space allotted. A light blue scroll bar has appeared on the right side of the pane. You are probably familiar with the concept of scrolling a window. In this program, each of the two panes can be scrolled separately.

Click on the small plus sign next to the finding "recently stopped medication" (highlighted in Figure 3-12). To scroll the nomenclature list, position the mouse pointer on the light blue scroll bar and hold the mouse button down while you drag the mouse in a downward motion. Continue scrolling the list until you can see all the findings under "recently stopped medication."

► Figure 3-12 **Expanded past history (scroll bar is circled in red).**

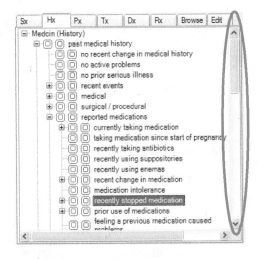

Step 4

Position the mouse pointer over the Sx tab and click the mouse once. The display will return to the previous list shown in Figure 3-8.

Position the mouse pointer over the small plus symbol for the finding "head-related symptoms" and click the mouse button. Notice the list fully expands to "chronic/recurring."

Step 5

Position the mouse pointer again over the Hx tab and click the mouse once. Notice the list is expanded as when you left it. In most cases, the software will remember how much of the expanded tree was displayed in each tab as well as what finding was highlighted. This feature allows the healthcare professional to easily go back to a previous tab to add another finding and then return where he or she left off.

Step 6

Explore each of the remaining sections of the Medcin nomenclature pane by clicking on each of the remaining tabs. Take a moment on each tab to look at the type of findings in that tab. Feel free to expand or collapse the list in any of the tabs.

Data Entry of Clinical Notes

The main purpose of EHR software such as those systems based on Medcin is to document clinical notes in a codified electronic medical record. This is done by selecting the finding from the Medcin nomenclature list in the left pane of the window. The finding and accompanying text are automatically recorded in the encounter note displayed in the right pane of the window. (The note view portion of the screen is indicated by the numeral 3 in Figure 3-3.)

Information is also added to the clinical note by adding or modifying a finding using the Entry Details fields in the bottom portion of the window. (The Entry Details section is indicated in Figure 3-3 by the numeral 4.)

The following exercises are designed to let you explore the interactions of the four sections of the Student Edition window. During the course of these exercises, you will create your first clinical encounter note with the Medcin nomenclature.

Guided Exercise 11: Creating an Encounter

When an outpatient visits a provider in a medical office or clinic, or when a provider examines a patient in a facility or at home, the meeting is commonly referred to as an *encounter*. Clinical notes documenting the encounter are variously referred to as *exam notes, provider notes,* or *encounter notes.* Whatever term is used, the encounter note is a record of the findings of an examination that occurred on a specific date and time. Although a portion of the data may be recorded by the medical assistant, another portion by the nurse, and yet another by a doctor, one completed encounter note should encompass the entire visit. If the patient returns for another visit, however, a new encounter is created.

In any type of medical facility, it is important to accurately record the date and time of the encounter. In this exercise, you will create a new encounter and learn how to set the date and time of the encounter.

Step 1

The name of the patient Carla Lopez should be displayed at the top of the Medcin window. If it is not, repeat Exercise 8.

The Select menu (which you have used previously) has functions for selecting an existing encounter or creating a new encounter. In this exercise, you will create a new encounter.

Position the mouse pointer over the word Select in the Menu bar, and click the mouse button. Move the mouse pointer vertically down the list until the item New Encounter is highlighted. Click the mouse button.

Step 2

When you create a new encounter, a window is invoked that allows you to set the date, time, and reason for the visit. The month, day, year, and time will default to current date and time settings in your own computer. Today's month and year are displayed in the calendar on the window. Today's date is outlined in red. Days that occur in the previous and subsequent months are in gray text.

Because it is unlikely that you are doing this exercise on May 1, 2012, you will need to manually set the date and time as instructed in this exercise. The purpose of this exercise is to teach you how to set the date and time using the New Encounter window.

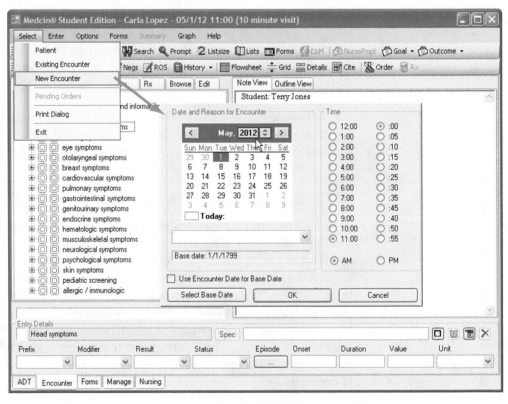

▶ Figure 3-13 **Date and time of new encounter: May 1, 2012 11:00 AM.**

Setting the Date to May 1, 2012 Small gray buttons with left and right arrows are located at the top of the calendar window. Clicking the button with the right arrow advances the calendar one month for each click of the mouse. Clicking the button with the left arrow takes the calendar backward one month for each click.

Click the buttons on the top of the calendar until the month "May" is displayed.

If the year 2012 is not currently displayed, click on the year to quickly modify it. Small buttons with up and down arrows will appear to the right of the year to allow you to quickly change years without cycling through all the months. Click the up or down arrow button to increase or decrease the year until 2012 is displayed.

Position the mouse pointer over day **1** and click the mouse button. The 1st will be highlighted with a blue rectangle.

The time is indicated on the right side of the window by white circles that are filled in with black centers. For example, in Figure 3-13, the circles next to 11:00 and :00 and AM are each filled, indicating the time of the encounter will be 11:00 AM.

Select the time by clicking your mouse in the circles next to "11:00" and ":00" and "AM." Each of the circles should become filled in.

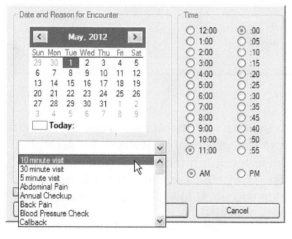

▶ **Figure 3-14 Select "10 minute visit" from the list of reasons for encounter.**

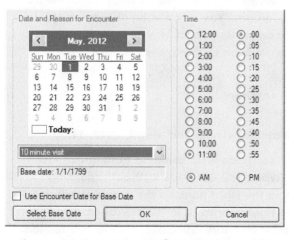

▶ **Figure 3-15 New encounter for a 10-minute visit, May 1, 2012 11:00 AM.**

Step 3

The reason for the encounter is also set in this window. The encounter Reason field is located just below the calendar. To view a list of reasons, position the mouse pointer over the button with the down arrow in the right side of the field, and click the mouse. A drop-down list of reasons will appear as shown in Figure 3-14.

Highlight the reason "10 minute visit" by moving the mouse pointer over it and then click the mouse button to select the reason.

Step 4

Compare your screen to Figure 3-15. Make certain you have set the date, time, and reason correctly. If the date, time, or reason needs to be corrected, repeat the previous steps.

Locate the button labeled OK in the bottom of the New Encounter window, position the mouse pointer over the OK button, and click the mouse. The "Date and Reason for Encounter" window will close.

Step 5

The encounter date, time, and reason (10 minute visit) should be displayed in the title of the window. The encounter date and time should be recorded in the encounter note in the right pane of the window.

Compare your screen with Figure 3-16; if your screen matches Figure 3-16, you are ready to proceed. If it does not, repeat steps 1 through 4 of this exercise.

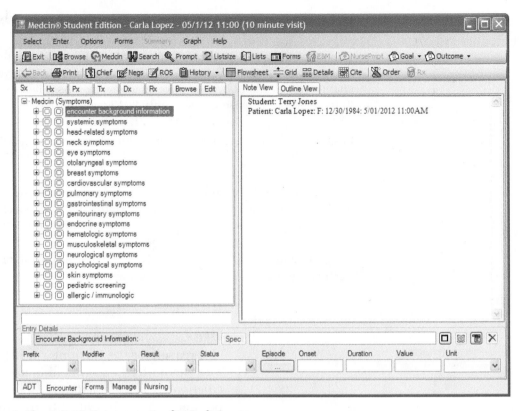

▶ Figure 3-16 New encounter for Carla Lopez.

Many of the exercises in subsequent chapters will permit you to use the current date and time and thus will not require this procedure. However, for several of the exercises, the date and time of the encounter must precisely match the date and time required for the exercise, in which case you will need this skill. Also, when working in a medical facility you must always record the date and time of the encounter accurately.

<table>
<tr><td>**Note**</td><td>**Tips for Completing the Exercises**</td></tr>
</table>

The purpose of this chapter is to help you become familiar with the software and EHR concepts through guided exercises. You will not be able to complete all of the exercises in this chapter in one class period. However, in subsequent class periods, each time you resume work on this chapter you must repeat at least three steps:

1. **Start the Medcin Student Edition software.**
2. **Select the patient, Carla Lopez.**
3. **Create a new encounter for a 10-minute visit dated May 1, 2012, 11:00 AM.**

In most cases, you will be able to continue with the next guided exercise without repeating preceding ones. When you continue without repeating prior exercises, the encounter note in the right pane of the window will not contain as much information as the figures printed in the textbook.

In Chapter 4 you will create and print an entire encounter note in one session.

Guided Exercise 12: Recording Subjective Findings

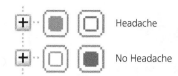

Headache

No Headache

▶ Figure 3-17 **Buttons adjacent to findings fill in with color when selected.**

Information is recorded in the encounter note by clicking the mouse on the buttons adjacent to each finding (shown enlarged in Figure 3-17). Clicking on a button with the red circle will record the finding as it appears in the list and fill in the red circle. Clicking on a button with the blue circle will record the finding in its opposite state and fill in the blue circle. For example, clicking on the button with the red circle next to headache will record that the patient has a headache; clicking on the button with the blue circle will record that the patient has reported no headache.

When a finding is recorded in the encounter note on the right pane, the description of the finding in the left pane also changes to match the selected state. For example, the finding "Headache" becomes "No Headache" when the blue button is selected, as shown in Figure 3-17.

Because the description of the findings change when their buttons are clicked, instructions to click a red or blue button identify a finding by its description *before* it is selected, so that you can locate it in the nomenclature pane. Screen figures used for comparison show the description of a finding as it appears *after* being selected.

For the remainder of this book, the buttons used to select findings will simply be referred to as the "red button" or the "blue button."

A finding can be highlighted (surrounded with a blue background) without selecting either the red or blue button by clicking on the description of the finding instead of the buttons. You will learn to highlight a finding later, in Exercise 19.

Step 1

Make sure that you have the Sx tab in the left pane selected. If you are uncertain, position the mouse pointer over the Sx tab and click the mouse once.

Using the skills you have acquired in a previous exercise, navigate the list of findings, and expand the tree of "head-related symptoms" until your list resembles the expanded tree shown in the left pane of Figure 3-18.

Step 2

Position the mouse over the red button for the finding "Headache." Click the mouse button. Compare your screen to Figure 3-18.

The center of the button should turn red. This indicates that the finding has been selected. The word "Headache" should have also appeared on the right pane in the encounter note.

When you record the first subjective finding, a section title "History of present illness" and the entry "Carla Lopez is a 27 year old female" are added to the encounter note as well.

Section titles are dynamically added or removed by the software based on the findings selected. This creates a nice looking encounter note without adding empty sections. For example, if tests are not ordered, the right pane does not show an empty section called "Tests."

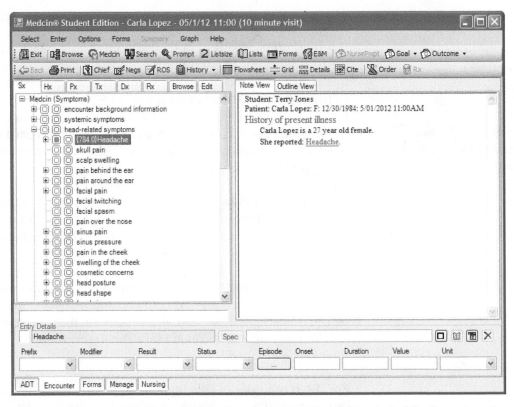

▶ Figure 3-18 **Expanded tree for "head-related symptoms" with "Headache" finding selected.**

Step 3

To further explore the operation of the red and blue buttons, position the mouse over and then click on the blue button for "Headache" instead. The center of the button should turn blue and the red button should return to its previous (cleared) state. Also the text in the encounter note and the finding description will both change to "No Headache."

Click on the red button to restore the finding back to "Headache." Make sure the button is red and the text in the encounter note again reads "Headache."

Step 4

EHR information should be as specific as possible. If the patient indicates that her headaches are chronic, you will want to select a more specific finding.

Click on the small plus next to "Headache" to expand the tree. Locate the finding "timing" and click the small plus next to it.

Locate the finding "chronic/recurring" and click on the red button.

Did the circle turn red? Did the text change in the encounter note?

Step 5

The patient further reports that her headaches have been getting worse.

Notice the small plus sign next to "chronic/recurring," which indicates that there are more detailed findings available. Click on the plus sign to expand the tree.

Compare your screen to Figure 3-19.

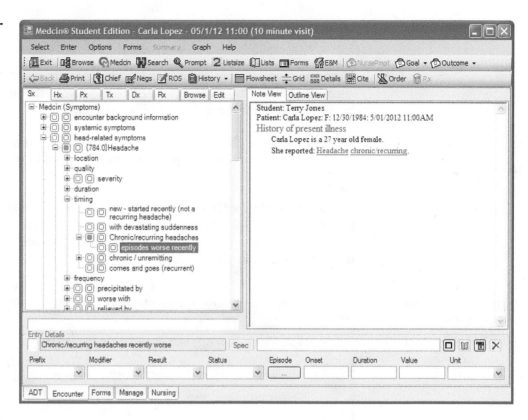

Step 6

In the expanded list for "chronic/recurring," click the mouse on the red button for "episodes worse recently."

Notice that the software changes the description of findings when you click a red or blue button to select them. In this case, the finding description changes to "chronic/recurring headaches recently worse." If the finding descriptions become too long, they are displayed truncated with an ellipsis (three dots), which indicates there is more to the description than will fit in the left pane.

Guided Exercise 13: Removing Findings

In step 3 of the previous exercise you learned that you could change the state or meaning of a finding that was already recorded by simply clicking your mouse on the opposite color button. In that example, clicking on the blue button changed "headache" to "no headache" and clicking on the red button changed it back to "headache."

However, what if you accidentally clicked on the wrong finding? How would you undo it completely? In this exercise, you will learn how to remove findings from the encounter note.

Step 1

As mentioned previously, the left pane has two additional tabs, Browse and Edit. In this exercise, we are going to use the Edit tab.

Look at the encounter note displayed in the right pane. Notice that findings in the encounter note are underlined and surrounding text is black. Section titles are blue text, but not underlined. You can click on underlined findings. You cannot click on section titles or the black text (i.e., you cannot click on text that is not underlined).

Move your mouse pointer over the underlined finding "with episodes" in the encounter note. The mouse pointer changes into the shape of a hand. While the hand is over the finding, click the mouse once. This will Edit the finding.

The Edit tab above the nomenclature pane has been automatically selected and the list in the nomenclature pane has been limited to the one finding being edited.

Step 2

Locate the button with an X in the lower right corner of the screen. (It is circled in red in Figure 3-20.) This is the Delete button, which is similar in appearance to the Delete button used in word processors, e-mail, and many other Windows programs. Position your mouse pointer over the Delete button and click once.

► Figure 3-20 **Edit mode and delete finding button (circled in red).**

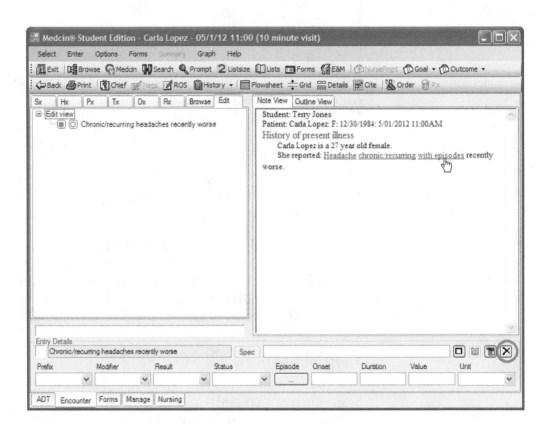

A small window called a dialogue will appear (as shown in Figure 3-21). The dialogue is asking you to confirm your intention to remove the finding from the encounter note.

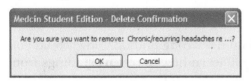

► Figure 3-21 **Click OK to confirm removing the finding.**

Note this procedure only removes the finding from the patient's current encounter note. Findings will not be deleted from the Medcin nomenclature or other patient encounters by this procedure.

Click on the OK button.

The finding "with episodes" and the text "recently worse" will be removed from the encounter note. The left pane will remain on the Edit tab. This is normal.

Step 3

Practice removing findings by repeating steps 1 and 2 for each of the other two findings: headaches and chronic/recurring. The order in which you remove them does not matter.

When you have removed the last finding for the section, the section title "History of present illness" and "Carla Lopez is a 27 year old female" will be removed automatically.

Step 4

Restore the Medcin nomenclature list to the left pane by positioning the mouse over the Sx tab and clicking once.

Guided Exercise 14: Recording More Specific Findings

In a previous exercise, you recorded a patient's symptom of chronic/recurring headaches by selecting three different findings from the list. There is nothing wrong with doing it that way if the natural flow of the exam progresses in that manner. For example, if when the patient reports having headaches and the clinician asks if they are recurring, the patient says "yes," the healthcare provider records the finding "recurring." Then, if the patient adds that they are getting worse, the provider adds the finding "worse."

However, if you have all of the information before selecting the finding, you can simply select the most specific finding and Medcin will add the hierarchical findings. In this exercise, you will record all three pieces of information about the patient's symptom by clicking only one finding.

Step 1

If your screen does not currently resemble Figure 3-16, repeat the necessary steps to select a patient, select a new encounter, and then select the Sx tab.

Expand the tree view of "head-related symptoms," "headache," "timing," and "chronic/recurring" (by clicking on the small plus signs) until you can see the full list shown in Figure 3-22.

Step 2

Position the mouse pointer over the red button for the finding "episodes recently worse" (indented under "chronic/recurring") and click the mouse.

Compare your screen with Figure 3-22. Did the circle in the button turn red?

Compare the text of the encounter note in Figure 3-22 with the text in Figure 3-20. The two notes read differently, but are medically equivalent. Additionally, in the codified EHR, Medcin has taken care of correlating the underlying codes.

In the real-world application of electronic medical records, speed of input is important. Use whichever technique accurately documents the exam in the least amount of time. There is no reason to go back and delete the findings as we did in the previous exercise when they are correct. However, when an entire symptom or observation can be documented by selecting a single finding, do so,

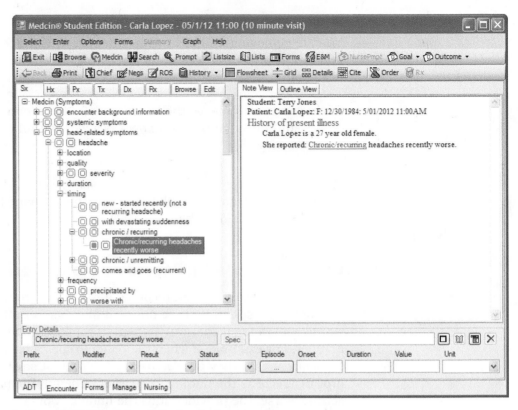

▶ Figure 3-22 **Chronic/recurring headaches recently worse.**

as you have in this exercise. The purpose of Exercise 13 was to teach you how to remove findings when necessary.

Guided Exercise 15: Recording History Findings

The History tab is used to record the patient's past medical, surgical, family, and social history.

Step 1

Position the mouse pointer over the Hx tab and click the mouse once.

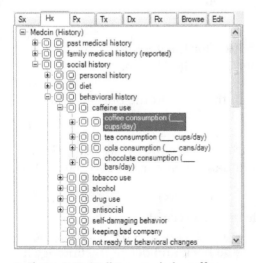

Step 2

Using the skills you have acquired in previous exercises, navigate the Medcin list, and expand the tree by clicking on the small plus signs next to "social history," "behavioral history," and "caffeine use." The left pane of the window should resemble Figure 3-23.

Step 3

Position the mouse over the red button next to the finding "coffee consumption (cups/day)." Click the mouse button. The circle in the button should turn red and "Behavioral: Daily coffee consumption" should appear in the encounter note pane on the right pane.

▶ Figure 3-23 **Hx list expanded—coffee consumption.**

Compare your screen to Figure 3-24. Note that two new titles were added as well, "Personal history" and "Behavioral."

▶ Figure 3-24 **Daily coffee consumption.**

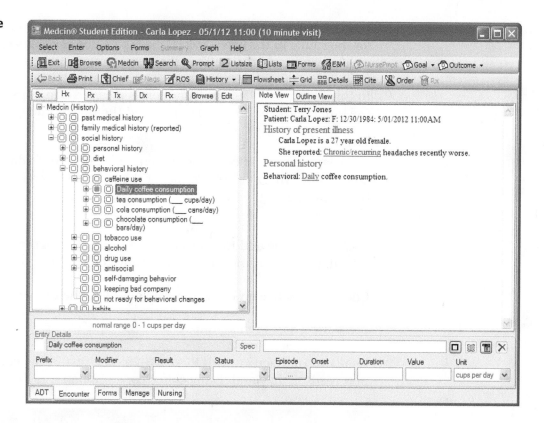

Adding Details to the Findings

In addition to the narrative text that the software automatically generates, you also can add further clarification to the encounter note using the Entry Details fields. The section labeled "Entry Details" is located at the bottom of your screen (identified in Figure 3-3 with the numeral 4).

The Entry Details section consists of two rows of white boxes. These are the Entry Details fields.

The first row of fields contains the description of the currently highlighted finding, a note field for adding free text about the current finding, and four buttons. You have already used the delete button (with the X) in a previous exercise. We will discuss and use the other buttons in later exercises.

The second row contains the following fields: Prefix, Modifier, Result, Status, Episode, Onset, Duration, Value, and Unit.

All of the fields in the Entry Details section apply to a single finding, the one currently selected.

In the following exercises you will learn to use the Entry Details fields. Notice the Entry Details fields as you select findings. In some cases, Medcin will automatically set one or more of the fields; in other cases you will set the field yourself.

Guided Exercise 16: Adding a Value

The Value field can be used to enter a value about any type of finding. For example, the patient's weight could be entered for a finding of weight, or the result of a simple blood test could be entered as a numeric value for the finding Hematocrit.

The Unit field is related to the Value field in that it describes the unit of measure for the value. In the two previous examples, the unit for weight would be pounds or kilograms, and the unit for the Hematocrit would be percent.

In this exercise, coffee consumption is measured in cups. So the value will be the number the patient consumed and the unit would be "cups per day."

Step 1

Make sure "Daily coffee consumption" is the current finding. If you are beginning a new class, you will need to repeat the previous exercise to add the finding before proceeding.

Step 2

Locate the Value and Unit fields in the Entry Details section at the bottom of the screen. Notice that the Unit field already contains the words "cups per day."

Click your mouse on the value field and type the numerals **7-8**.

Press the Enter key on your keyboard.

Compare your screen with Figure 3-25. The text in the encounter note should now read: "Behavioral: Daily coffee consumption was 7-8 cups per day."

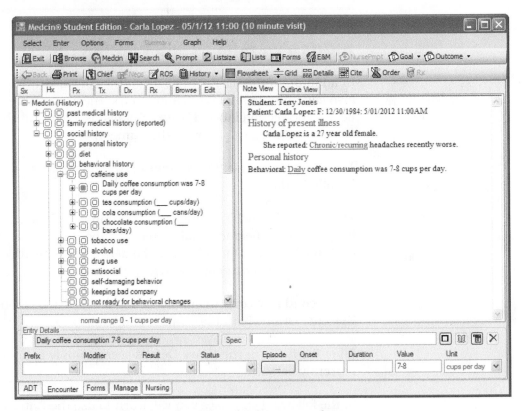

▶ Figure 3-25 **Recording the value, 7-8, and Unit, cups per day.**

Using Free Text

In this exercise you will learn how to add your own text into the note. The term for this is *free text*, meaning that the text is not codified and can contain anything.

In contrast, the other Entry Details fields (Prefix, Modifier, Result, Status, Episode, Onset, Duration, Value, and Unit) are stored as fielded data. Remember, fielded data has the advantage of producing a uniform, searchable EHR.

Ideally the less free text used in the EHR the better. Still, oftentimes free text is appropriate, for example, when adding a nuance to a finding that extends its meaning or entering text to portray the patient's own words more accurately.

Guided Exercise 17: Adding Free Text

In this exercise, the patient reports she has recently stopped drinking coffee.

Step 1

Click on the small plus sign next to "Daily coffee consumption" to expand the list of findings. If you are beginning a new class, you will need to repeat the two previous exercises to add the finding before proceeding.

Locate the finding "recently decreased" and click the mouse on the red button. Compare your screen to Figure 3-26.

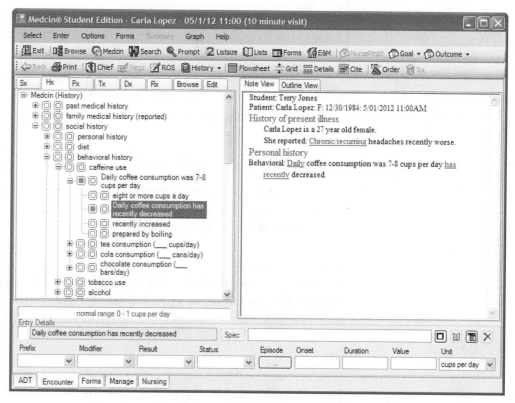

▶ Figure 3-26 **Patient reported decreased coffee consumption.**

Step 2

Look at the Entry Details section at the bottom of your screen. There are two long fields in the first row. The gray field on the left contains the description that appears in the note and cannot be directly edited; the field on the right is used to add free text to the currently selected finding.

Click your mouse in the free-text field. Type **because she stopped all coffee** in the field and then press the Enter key on your keyboard. Compare your screen with Figure 3-27.

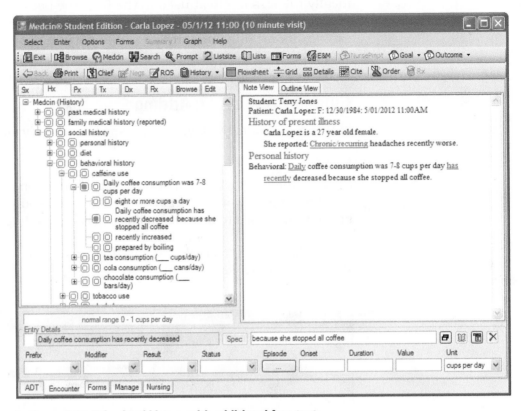

▶ Figure 3-27 **Behavioral history with additional free text.**

Guided Exercise 18: Recording Objective Findings

The Px tab is used to record the observations and results of the clinician's physical examination of the patient as well as the measurements called vital signs recorded by the medical assistant.

Step 1

Position the mouse pointer over the Px tab and click the mouse once. The Physical Examination list will be displayed. Notice that the list is organized by body systems, essentially in the order you would perform a head-to-toe exam.

Step 2

Click on the small plus sign next to "Head" to expand the list. Locate the finding "Exam for evidence of injury" and click the mouse on the blue button. Compare your screen to Figure 3-28. The blue button should be filled in and the text "No evidence of a head injury" should be recorded in the encounter note pane.

Step 3

Look at the Entry Details field for Result. It was previously blank but now contains the word "normal." This is an example of how the EHR software can set the field for you based on the assumption that it is normal not to have a head injury.

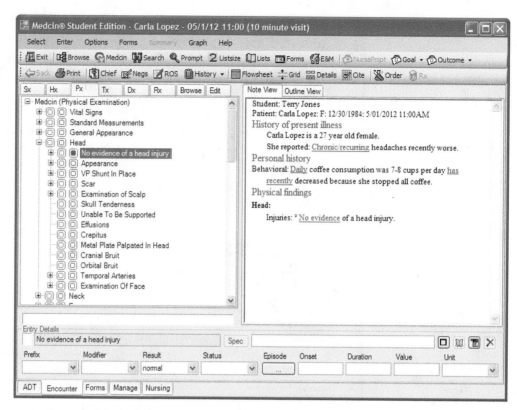

▶ Figure 3-28 **No head injury.**

Guided Exercise 19: Setting the Result Field

As mentioned earlier, the software can set Entry Detail fields automatically (as in the previous exercise) or you can set the field. In this exercise you will learn how to highlight a finding and how to set the Result field.

Step 1

Using the mouse, scroll the list of physical examination findings until you see Neurological System. Expand the list by clicking on the small plus sign next to Neurological System.

Step 2

Locate the finding "Cognitive Functions" and highlight the finding by clicking your mouse on the description (not on the red or blue buttons). Compare your screen to Figure 3-29.

Step 3

The Prefix, Modifier, Result, Status, and Unit fields have buttons next to the field with an arrow pointing down. This type of button indicates there is a drop-down list of items you can choose for that field. You have previously used this type of list to select the reason when creating a new encounter.

Locate the Result field in the Entry Details section at the bottom of the screen. Click your mouse on the button with the down arrow in the field. A drop-down list of choices (as shown in Figure 3-30) will appear. Do not be concerned if the software positions a drop-down list differently from the positions shown in the figures in this book. Drop-down lists may appear either above or below a field, depending on the screen settings of each computer.

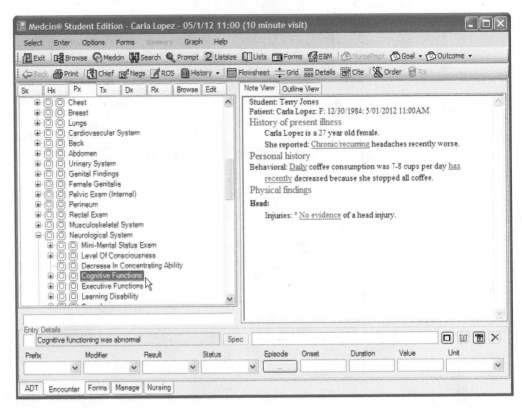

▶ Figure 3-29 Neurological System/Cognitive Functions finding highlighted.

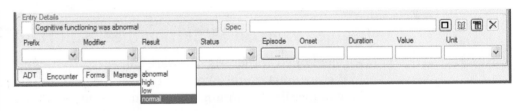

▶ Figure 3-30 Drop-down list for Result field.

Position your mouse pointer on the result "normal" and click the mouse button. The field will display the word "normal," the blue button will have automatically been selected, and the encounter note will read "Cognitive functioning was normal."

Guided Exercise 20: Adding Detail to Recorded Findings

EHR software must be very flexible because additional observations or information from the patient could necessitate going back to any section at any time. In this exercise, you will add status information to the patient's reported symptom.

Step 1

Select the finding for edit by moving your mouse pointer over the words "Chronic/recurring" (in the headache entry) in the right pane. When the mouse pointer changes to a hand; click the mouse button. The Px tab in the left pane should be replaced by the Edit tab. This step of the procedure is the same one you used in Exercise 13 to remove findings.

"Chronic/recurring headache" is now the current finding.

Step 2

Locate the Status field in the Entry Details section at the bottom of the screen. Click your mouse on the button with the down arrow in the status field. A drop-down list of phrases (as shown in Figure 3-31) will appear.

► Figure 3-31 **Drop-down list for Status field.**

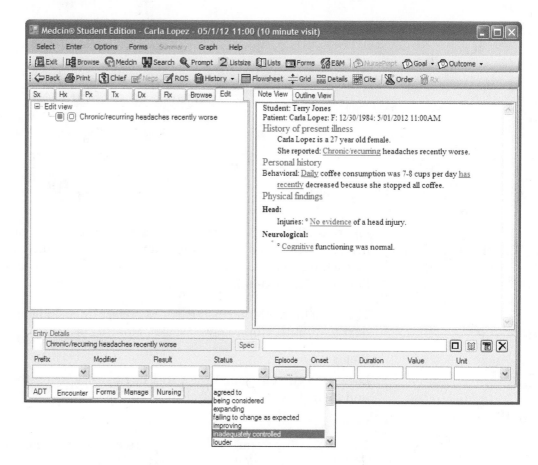

Step 3

Position your mouse pointer on the status "inadequately controlled" and click the mouse button. The field will display a portion of the phrase, and the text in the encounter note will change to "Chronic/recurring headaches recently worse which is inadequately controlled."

Guided Exercise 21: Adding Episode Detail to Findings

In addition to drop-down lists, another method of input allows you to quickly enter numerical data. In this exercise, you will add information about the frequency of the patient's headaches.

Step 1

The finding "Chronic/recurring" in the headache entry should still be selected for edit. If it is not, then repeat step 1 of the previous exercise.

Step 2

Locate the label "Episode" in the Entry Details section at the bottom of your screen. The Episode button located below the label has an ellipsis (three dots) on it. Click your mouse on the Episode button. The Episode window shown in Figure 3-32 will be invoked. It is used to record information about the intervals and repetitions at which findings occur.

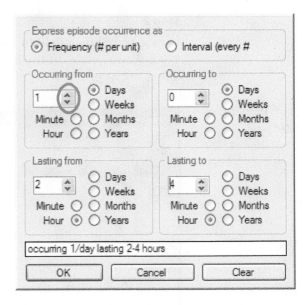

▶ Figure 3-32 **Episode window (numeric controls circled in red.)**

Figure 3-32 has a red circle drawn around the control buttons for the numeric fields. Increase or decrease the numeric value of a field in the Episode window by clicking on the up or down arrow buttons next to the numeric field (circled in red in Figure 3-32).

The units in which time is measured are set by clicking on one of the white circles next to Minute, Hour, Days, Weeks, Months, or Years.

Step 3

Locate "Occurring from." Set it to 1 day by clicking on the up arrow button once and then clicking on the circle next to Days.

Step 4

Locate "Lasting from." Set it to 2 hours by clicking on the up arrow button twice and then clicking on the circle next to Hour.

Step 5

Locate "Lasting to." Set it to 4 hours by clicking on the up arrow button four times and then clicking on the circle next to Hour.

Step 6

Compare your screen to the Episode window in Figure 3-32, and then click on the OK button.

Look at the encounter note in the right pane. Does the text read "Chronic/recurring headaches recently worse occurring 1/day lasting 2–4 hours which is inadequately controlled"?

Guided Exercise 22: Recording the Assessment

The assessment is the clinician's diagnosis of the patient's problem or condition. This exercise will give you further experience in navigating and expanding the *tree* of findings.

Step 1

Position your mouse pointer on the tab "Dx" and click the mouse. The Diagnosis, Syndromes, and Conditions list should be displayed in the left pane of the window.

Step 2

Scroll down the list until you see "Neurologic Disorders" (highlighted in Figure 3-33.) Click on the small plus sign to expand the list.

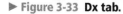 ▶ Figure 3-33 **Dx tab.**

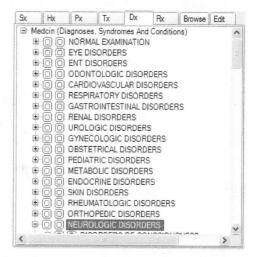

Locate "Headache Syndromes" in the list and click on the small plus sign.

Step 3

Scroll the list further downward until you see "Benign Syndromes" (highlighted in Figure 3-34) and then click on the small plus sign.

▶ Figure 3-34 **Dx tab scrolled to Benign Syndromes.**

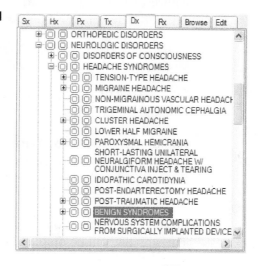

Step 4

Scroll further down the list until you see "Drug-Induced Headache" and then click on the small plus sign.

Step 5

Scroll further down the list until you see "Vasoconstrictor withdrawal headache" and then click on the small plus sign.

The fully expanded list of findings is shown in Figure 3-35.

Step 6

Position your mouse pointer on the red button next to "From caffeine" and click the mouse. Compare your screen to Figure 3-35. The finding "Vasoconstrictor

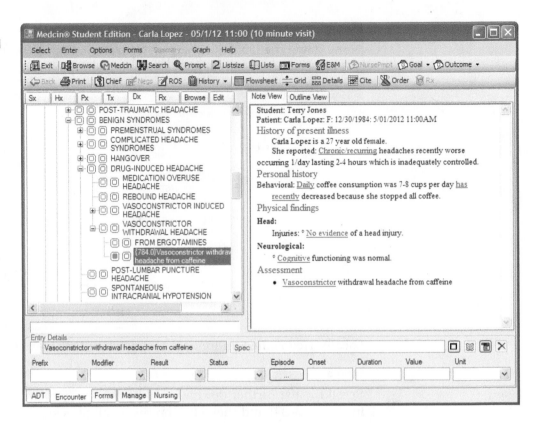

withdrawal headache from caffeine" should be recorded in the encounter note under a new heading, Assessment.

Guided Exercise 23: Recording Treatment Plan and Physician Orders

In Exercise 12, you added free text to a specific finding. Medcin also has several special findings that are used as anchors for general free-text entry.

Additionally, when you have more than a few words of free text to enter, a larger window may be useful as well. In this exercise, you will add a free-text finding and enter information through a special free-text window.

Step 1

Position the mouse pointer on the Rx tab and click the mouse button. The Medcin Therapy list will be displayed.

Step 2

Scroll to the bottom of the list and locate the finding labeled "Free Text" as shown in Figure 3-36.

Highlight the finding "Free Text" (not the red or blue button).

Step 3

This time, instead of typing free text into the Entry Details field, you will invoke a small window used for adding and editing finding notes. In the lower right corner of your screen are four buttons. You used the delete button (with the X) in previous exercises. In this exercise you will use the Finding Note button, which is circled in red in Figure 3-37.

Position your mouse pointer on the Finding Note button and click the mouse. A small Finding Note window will be invoked as shown in Figure 3-37.

► Figure 3-36 **Locate free-text finding on Rx tab.**

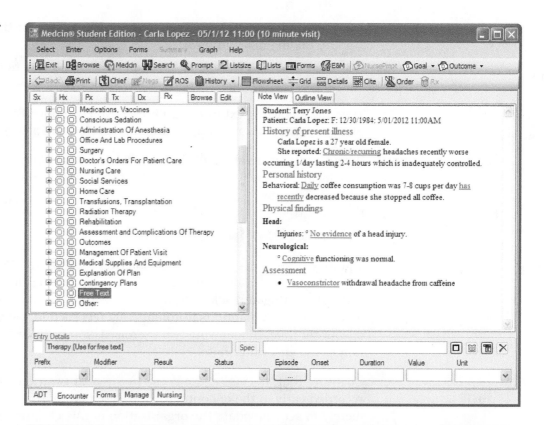

► Figure 3-37 **Finding Note window used for free text (button circled in red.)**

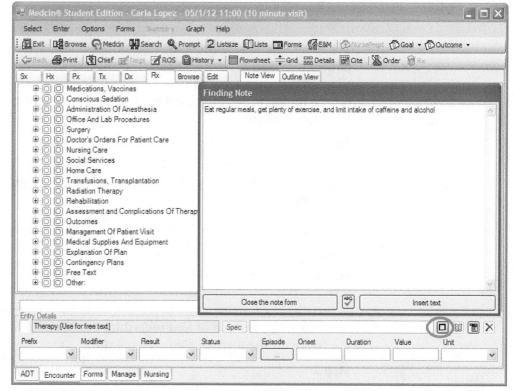

Step 4

There are several advantages to entering free text in this window as opposed to in the free-text field in the Entry Details section:

1. The area in the window is larger than the free-text field, making it easier to type longer notes.

2. The window includes a spell checker (the button at the bottom center of the finding note window).

3. The Insert text feature allows frequently used text to be stored and inserted as free text whenever appropriate, saving time typing.

Type the following text into the Finding Note window: **Eat regular meals, get plenty of exercise, and limit intake of caffeine and alcohol.**

When you have finished, click your mouse on the button labeled "Close the note form." This will add your text to the encounter note under a new section labeled "Therapy."

Introduction to Using Forms

You may have noticed in the previous exercise that the Finding Note window was called a *form*. Forms make it convenient to enter findings and free text without locating and selecting the finding from the nomenclature. When a form is used, the information is automatically recorded in the proper section of the encounter note. In following two exercises, you will use forms to add information to the encounter note.

Be aware that, normally, the items in the next two exercises would have been recorded early in the encounter; they were placed at the end of the exercises merely to accommodate the organization of this chapter.

Guided Exercise 24: Recording the Chief Complaint

Typically, the first thing recorded in the encounter is a description of the patient's reason for the visit. This is called the *chief complaint*. You could locate the finding "chief complaint" and then enter a free-text note, but because the chief complaint is a standard part of every exam, it is more efficient to use a form for text entry.

Step 1

As previously discussed, at the top of your screen are two rows of buttons called the Toolbar. The purpose of the Toolbar is to allow quick access to commonly used functions.

Locate the button in the Toolbar labeled "Chief" (circled in Figure 3-38.)

Step 2

Position your mouse pointer over the "Chief" button and click your mouse button. The Chief complaint window will be invoked. This window looks similar to the Finding Note window in the previous exercise except that when you close the note form, instead of just recording free text, it will automatically associate the text with the finding "Chief complaint."

Step 3

Type the following text into the finding note window: **Headaches for more than 5 days.**

When you have finished, compare your screen to Figure 3-38.

Position your mouse on the button labeled "Close the note form" and click the mouse. This will add a new section to the encounter note titled "Chief complaint" followed by the text you typed.

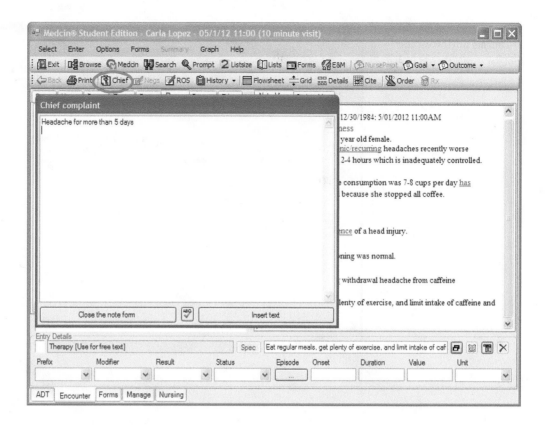

Guided Exercise 25: Recording Vital Signs

Forms are not limited to free text. Many findings can be included on one form, and the form can contain specific Entry Details fields such as Result, Status, Value, and Unit.

A form is frequently used to record vital signs (routine measurements of the body taken at nearly every medical practice). As you will see in this exercise, it is more efficient to enter numerical data using a form than to locate and select findings one at a time and then enter data in the Value field for each.

Step 1

At the very bottom of the screen are five tabs labeled ADT, Encounter, Forms, Manage, and Nursing. All forms except the small free-text boxes used in previous exercises are accessed from the Forms tab.

Position your mouse pointer over the tab labeled "Forms" (circled in red at the bottom of Figure 3-39) and click the mouse.

When the tab is clicked, the familiar encounter view in the right pane will be replaced with an Outline View of the headings that have findings in your encounter note. The Outline View presents the headings as icons of file folders, with small plus signs preceding them. If you click on a small plus sign, the tree will expand to show the findings recorded in the encounter under that heading. The Outline View will also show the ICD-9-CM and CPT-4 codes for relevant findings. Those codes will be discussed in Chapter 8.

Because you may not have performed all of the previous exercises in a single class period, your Outline View may not have as much detail as shown in Figure 3-39.

► Figure 3-39 **Forms tab and Forms button on the Toolbar (both circled in red).**

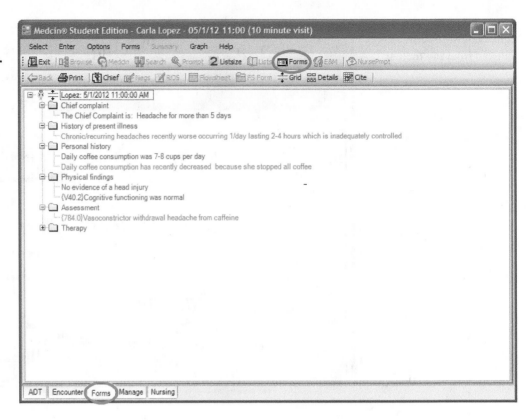

Step 2

Locate and click on the button labeled "Forms" in the top row of the Toolbar at the top of your screen. (The button is circled in red in Figure 3-39). This will invoke the Forms Manager window shown in Figure 3-40. The Forms Manager lists forms used in the Student Edition.

► Figure 3-40 **Select vitals from the list in the Forms Manager window.**

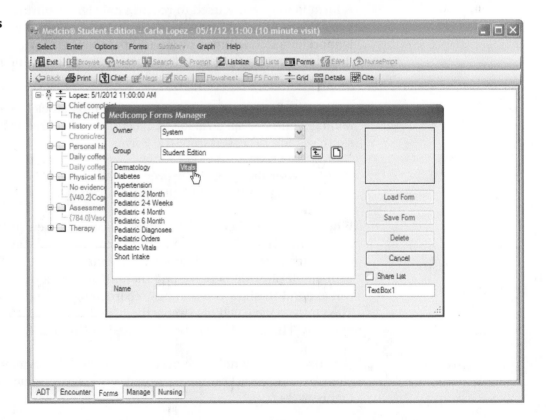

Locate and click on the form labeled "Vitals" in the Forms Manager window as shown in Figure 3-40. This should open the form shown in Figure 3-41.

▶ Figure 3-41 **Vitals form for Carla Lopez, with Encounter tab circled in red.**

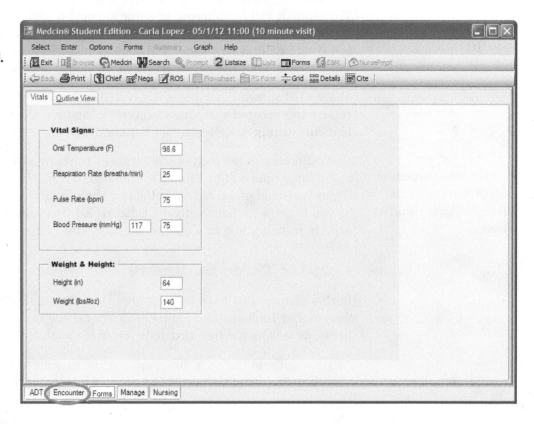

Enter Ms. Lopez's vital signs into the corresponding fields. They are as follows:

Temperature:	**98.6**
Respiration:	**25**
Pulse:	**75**
BP	**117/75**
Height:	**64**
Weight:	**140**

When you have entered all of the vital signs, compare your screen to Figure 3-41 and then click your mouse on the Encounter tab (circled in red) at the bottom of the screen.

The vital signs information will now be recorded in the encounter note on the right pane under the Physical Findings section.

Step 3

Look at the results of the vital signs entry as they appear in the encounter note. Also notice that there is a tab on top of the right pane labeled "Outline View." This tab will display the same outline in the right pane as was displayed on the Forms tab.

When you have finished looking at the note, exit the Student Edition software.

> **Note**
>
> **Systolic and diastolic blood pressure readings are entered in two separate fields. Omit the "/" character when entering blood pressure (BP) in the form.**

Visually Different Button Styles

The Medcin Student Edition software has been specially created for this course. Therefore, it will be different in some aspects from EHR systems you will encounter when working in a medical facility, but the concepts, skills, and familiarity with EHR systems you will acquire by practicing with the Student Edition will transfer directly into the workplace.

Many EHR software packages are based on the Medcin nomenclature. Each vendor has created a unique visual style, and although they share a common nomenclature, the EHR may look quite different.

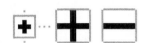

▶ Figure 3-42 **Alternative style of buttons used to select findings in some EHR systems.**

One difference is the look of the buttons. In many systems, a large plus sign and a large minus sign similar to those shown in Figure 3-42 are used to select findings instead of the red and blue buttons used in the Student Edition. However, as you become familiar with the Student Edition software, you should have no trouble transitioning to a similar Medcin-based EHR in your job.

Chapter Three Summary

In this chapter you have learned about the Student Edition software: the menus and Toolbar, the nomenclature pane, the note pane, the Entry Details fields, as well as the free-text note, chief complaint, and vital signs forms.

As you continue through the course, you can refer to the guided exercises in this chapter when you need to remember how to perform a particular task.

Task	Guided Exercise(s)	Page #
Starting up and exiting the software	6 and 7	47, 50
Select a patient	8	50
Navigating Medcin findings and tabs	9 and 10	52, 55
Creating an encounter by setting the date, time, and reason for visit	11	57
Recording findings		
Subjective findings	12	61
History findings	15	66
Objective findings	18	70
Assessment	22	74
Treatment plan	23	76
Removing findings or selecting findings to edit	13	63
Adding details to the findings		
Adding a value	16	67
Adding free text	17	69
Adding free text using the Finding Note window	23	76
Setting the Result field	19	71
Adding detail to recorded findings	20	72
Adding episode detail to findings	21	73
Using the Chief Complaint form	24	78
Using the Forms tab, Forms Manager, and Vitals form	25	79

Testing Your Knowledge of Chapter 3

You may run the Medcin Student Edition software and use your mouse on the screen to answer the following questions:

1. Which menu did you use to select the patient?

2. Which menu did you use to start a new encounter?

3. Where did you set the label "10 minute visit," which appeared in the title of the window?

The tabs in the Medcin Nomenclature pane have medical abbreviations. Write the meaning of each of the following:

4. Sx _____

5. Hx _____

6. Px _____

7. Tx _____

8. Dx _____

9. Rx _____

10. What was Carla Lopez's chief complaint?

11. Where in the Entry Details section did you record the frequency and duration of her headaches?

12. What was the clinical assessment (her diagnosis)?

13. How did you invoke the Vitals window?

14. How do you remove a finding?

15. How did you invoke the Chief Complaint window?

Increased Familiarity with the Software

Learning Outcomes

After completing this chapter, you should be able to:

- Create a new encounter
- Document a patient visit
- Print a copy of the completed encounter note

Applying Your Knowledge

In this chapter, you will practice documenting patient encounters using the Student Edition software. One of the goals in this chapter is to increase your familiarity with the software and thereby increase your speed of data entry. Another is to learn how to print your work.

The encounter notes you will produce will be similar to documents you would create in a medical facility. Exercises in this chapter are intended to provide conceptual learning experiences with the software; however, they are not intended to represent full and complete medical exams.

In Chapter 3, you learned the basic layout of the screen and the concepts of creating an encounter note, adding and editing findings, and adding details to findings. Detailed instructions for scrolling and navigating the lists, which were provided in the previous chapter, should no longer be necessary. From this point forward, simplified instructions will guide you in areas where you are already familiar with the program. Also, red or blue circles will be printed in the text as a visual cue to indicate whether to click on a red or blue button to select a finding.

One important point to remember is that the Student Edition software does **not** save your entries into the patient's permanent medical record; therefore, you will **keep a record of your work by printing it.** Whereas in the previous chapter you could stop exercises at any time, from this point forward it is important to complete the entire exercise and print out your work before stopping. In the next two exercises you will learn how to use the print function.

You can print the encounter note at any time and as often as you like while practicing your exercises. However, remember not to quit or exit the program **until you are sure the encounter note has printed.** Once you exit, you will lose your work.

Creating Your First Patient Encounter Note

In Exercise 26, you will apply what you learned in Chapter 3 to document Carla Lopez's visit. In Exercise 27, you will print out your work to hand in to your instructor. You must complete both exercises in a single session. Do not begin Exercise 26 unless you have enough class time remaining to complete both exercises.

Guided Exercise 26: Documenting a Visit for Headaches

Carla Lopez visits her doctor's office complaining of headaches for the last 5 days. The exercise is similar, but not identical to the cumulative exercises in Chapter 3.

Step 1

If you have not already done so, start the Student Edition software.

Locate the Medcin icon shown in Chapter 3, Figure 3-1. If you do not see it on the computer desktop, click on the Start button, and look in Programs or All Programs for the program named Medcin SE.

Step 2

When the Student Edition login screen is displayed, type into the field either your name or student ID (whichever is preferred by your instructor).

When your name or ID is exactly as you want it to be, position the mouse pointer over the button labeled "OK," and click the mouse. The Student Edition software window will be displayed.

Step 3

Position the mouse pointer over the word Select in the menu at the top of the screen and click the mouse button once. A list of the Select menu options will appear.

Click the mouse on the word Patient to invoke the Patient Selection window shown in Figure 4-1.

Select the patient named "Carla Lopez."

► Figure 4-1 **Select Carla Lopez from Patient Selection window.**

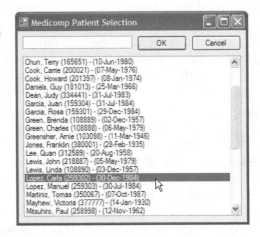

Step 4

Again, position the mouse pointer over the word Select, and click the mouse button. Move the mouse pointer vertically down the list until the item New Encounter is highlighted. Click the mouse button.

Using what you have learned in previous exercises, from the Select menu, click New Encounter. Then select the reason **10 minute visit** from the drop-down list.

You may use the current date; you do not have to set the date or time for this exercise. However, be certain to set the encounter reason correctly.

Compare the reason field on your screen to that shown in Figure 4-2 before clicking on the OK button.

► Figure 4-2 **New Encounter set for a "10 minute visit."**

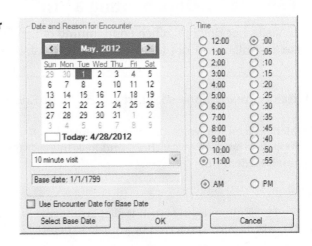

The left pane should display the Medcin Symptoms list and the right pane should display your student ID and Carla Lopez's information. Before proceeding, confirm that the patient and the reason for the visit displayed in the title of the window are all correct.

Step 5

Enter the chief complaint by locating the button in the Toolbar labeled "Chief" and clicking on it.

The Chief complaint window will open. Type **Headaches for more than 5 days**.

Compare your screen to Figure 4-3. If it is correct, click the button labeled "Close the note form."

▶ Figure 4-3 **Chief complaint: Headaches for more than 5 days.**

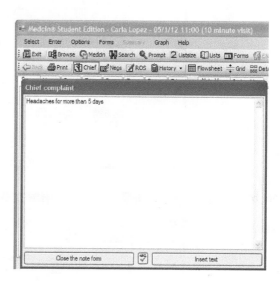

Step 6

Make sure that you have the Sx tab in the left pane selected. If you are uncertain, position the mouse pointer over the Sx tab and click the mouse once. Using the skills you have acquired in previous exercises, navigate the list of findings.

Locate and expand the tree of head-related symptoms.

Click on the small plus sign next to "head-related symptoms."

Click on the small plus sign next to "headache."

Click on the small plus sign next to "timing."

Click on the small plus sign next to "chronic/recurring."

Locate and click on the red button next to the following finding:

● (red button) episodes worse recently

Compare your screen to Figure 4-4.

Step 7

Add information about the episodes of Ms. Lopez's headaches by scrolling the nomenclature pane to show more of the findings under the expanded tree of headache symptoms:

► Figure 4-4 **Sx tab: chronic recurring headaches recently worse.**

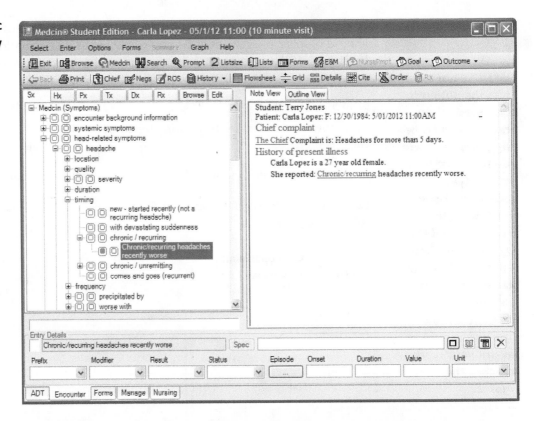

► Figure 4-5 **Set frequency to "Daily."**

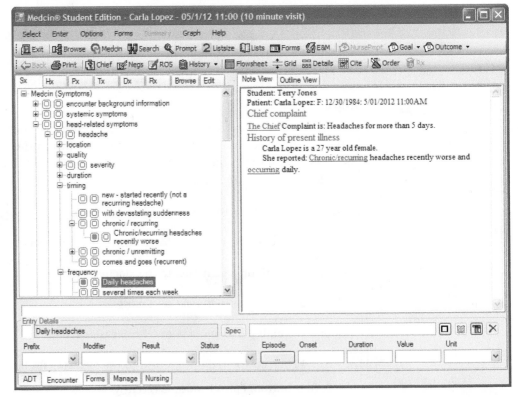

Locate and click on the small plus sign next to "frequency."

Locate and click on the red button next to the following finding:

● (red button) daily

Compare your screen to Figure 4-5.

Step 8

Select the finding "Chronic/recurring" for edit by moving your mouse pointer over the words "Chronic/recurring" headache in the encounter note pane on the right. When the mouse pointer changes to a hand, click the mouse button. The Sx tab in the left pane should be replaced by the Edit tab with "Chronic/recurring headaches recently worse" as the current finding.

Step 9

Locate the Status field in the Entry Details section at the bottom of the screen. Click your mouse on the button with the down arrow in the status field. A drop-down list of status phrases (as shown in Figure 4-6) will appear.

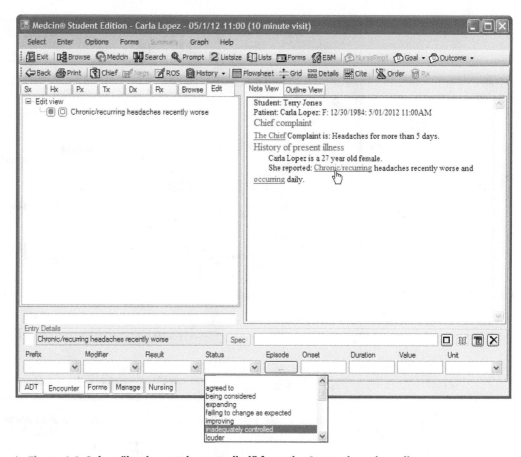

▶ Figure 4-6 **Select "inadequately controlled" from the Status drop-down list.**

Position your mouse pointer on the status "inadequately controlled" and click the mouse button.

Step 10

Position the mouse pointer over the Hx tab and click the mouse once.

Locate and expand the social history tree, by clicking on the small plus sign next to "social history."

Click on the small plus sign next to "behavioral history."

Click on the small plus sign next to "caffeine use."

Locate and click on the red button next to the following finding:

- (red button) coffee consumption (cups/day)

Step 11

Locate the Value and Unit fields in the Entry Details section at the bottom of the screen. Notice that the Unit field already contains the words "cups per day."

Click your mouse on the Value field and type the numerals **7-8**.

Press the Enter key on your keyboard.

Compare your screen to Figure 4-7.

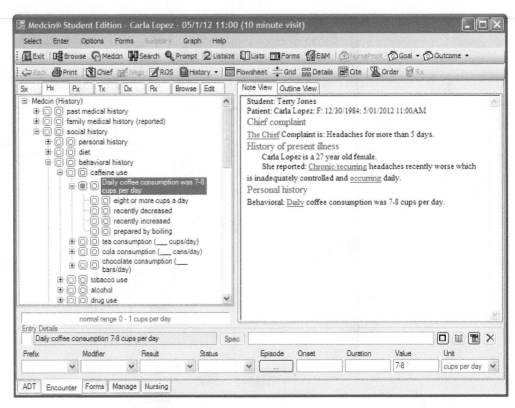

▶ **Figure 4-7 Social history: Daily coffee consumption was 7-8 cups per day.**

Step 12

In the left pane, click on the small plus sign next to "Daily coffee consumption." This will expand the tree.

Locate and click on the red button next to the following finding:

- (red button) recently decreased

Step 13

Locate the free-text field in the first row of the Entry Details section, under the right pane.

Click your mouse in the free-text field. Type **because she stopped all coffee** in the field and then press the Enter key on your keyboard. Compare your screen with Figure 4-8.

► **Figure 4-8 Caffeine recently decreased because she stopped all coffee.**

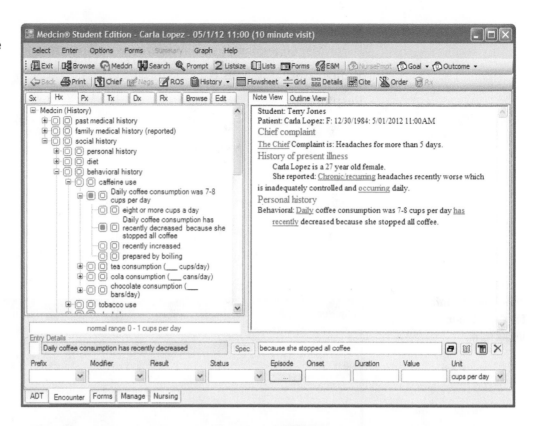

► **Figure 4-9 Select "Vitals" from Forms Manager window (Forms button circled in red).**

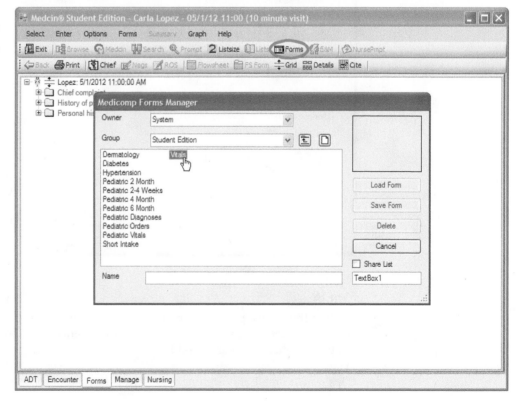

Step 14

Locate and click on the button labeled "Forms" in the top row of buttons on the Toolbar. The tabs at the bottom of the screen will automatically change to the Form tab. The Forms Manager window will be invoked.

Locate and double-click on the form labeled Vitals (see Figure 4-9).

Step 15

Enter Ms. Lopez's vital signs into the corresponding fields as follows:

Temperature: **98.6**

Respiration: **25**

Pulse: **75**

BP: **117/75**

Height: **64**

Weight: **140**

When you have entered all of the vital signs, compare your screen to Figure 4-10 and then click your mouse on the Encounter tab at the bottom of the screen.

▶ Figure 4-10 **Information for Carla Lopez entered in Vitals form.**

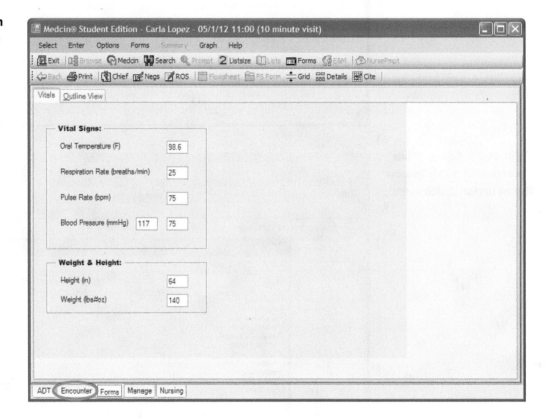

Step 16

Position the mouse pointer over the Px tab and click the mouse once. Notice that the vital signs information has been recorded in the encounter note under the Physical Findings section (see Figure 4-11).

Click on the small plus sign next to "Head" to expand the list.

Locate and click on the blue button next to the following finding:

● (blue button) Exam for evidence of injury

Step 17

Using the mouse, scroll the list of physical examination findings until you see Neurological System. Expand the list by clicking on the small plus sign next to Neurological System.

► Figure 4-11 **Px tab: No evidence of a head injury.**

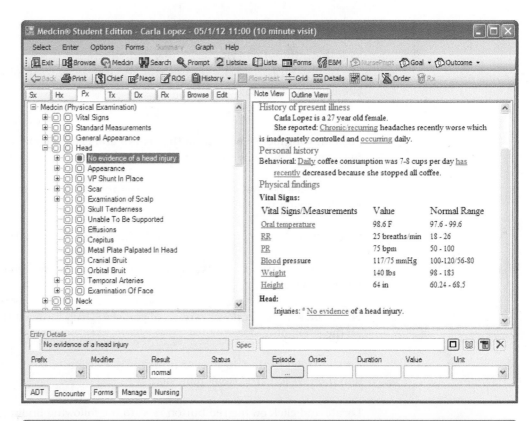

► Figure 4-12 **Px tab: Cognitive Functions normal.**

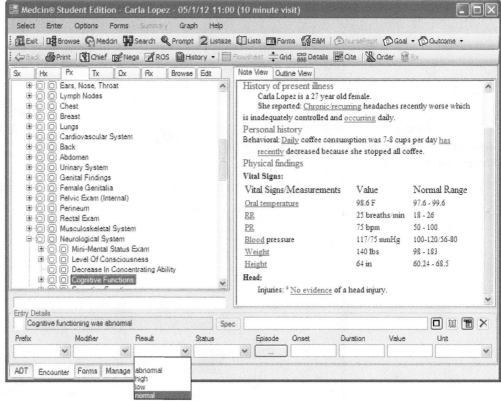

Locate and highlight the finding "Cognitive Functions" by clicking your mouse on the description. Do not click either the red or blue button.

Locate the Result field in the Entry Details section at the bottom of the screen. Click your mouse on the down arrow button within the Result field. A drop-down list will appear (as shown in Figure 4-12).

Position your mouse pointer on the result "normal" and click the mouse button.

The Result field will display the word "normal," the button next to the finding should be blue, and the text in the encounter note should read "Cognitive functioning was normal."

Step 18

Position your mouse pointer on the Dx tab and click the mouse. The Diagnosis, Syndromes, and Conditions list should be displayed in the left pane of the window.

Scroll the list downward until you see "Neurological Disorders." Click on the small plus sign to expand the list.

Locate "Headache Syndromes" in the list and click on the small plus sign.

Scroll the list further downward until you see "Benign Syndromes" and then click on the small plus sign.

Scroll the list further downward until you see "Drug-Induced Headache" and then click on the small plus sign.

Scroll the list further downward until you see "Vasoconstrictor withdrawal headache" and then click on the small plus sign.

Locate and click on the red button next to the following finding:

● (red button) from caffeine

Compare your screen to Figure 4-13. The finding "Vasoconstrictor withdrawal headache from caffeine" should be recorded in the encounter note under a new heading, "Assessment."

▶ Figure 4-13 **Dx tab: Assessment: vasoconstrictor withdrawal headache from caffeine.**

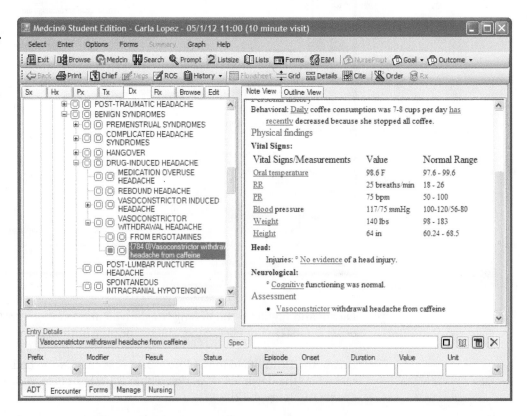

Step 19

Position the mouse pointer on the Rx tab and click the mouse button. The Medcin Therapy list will be displayed.

Scroll the list to locate and then click on the red button next to the following finding:

● (red button) Free Text

Locate and click on the Finding Note button (circled in red in the lower right corner of Figure 4-14). The Finding Note window will be invoked.

Type the following text into the Finding Note window: **Eat regular meals, drink ample water, and avoid caffeine and alcohol for one week.**

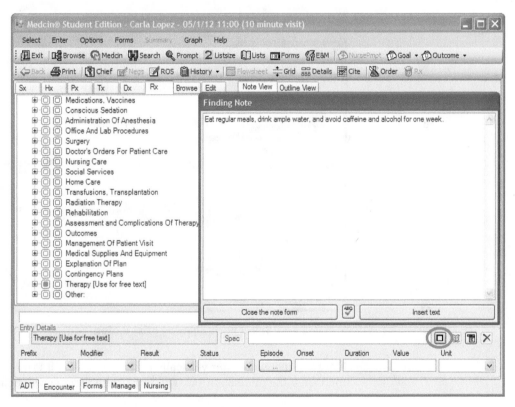

► Figure 4-14 **Rx tab: free-text Therapy finding note.**

When you have finished, compare your screen to Figure 4-14. If it matches, click your mouse on the button labeled "Close the note form." This will add your text to the encounter note.

You have now successfully created your first complete encounter note. However, do not stop or close the program until you complete the following exercise.

Guided Exercise 27: Printing the Encounter Note

The Student Edition software does **not** save your entries to the patient's permanent medical record; therefore, you will **keep a record of your work by printing it.** In this exercise, you will learn to print the encounter note. You will be asked to give your finished printout to your instructor.

You can use either of two methods to print your work: You can print to a printer
or to a file. The method you will use will be based on the policy of your school.
Your instructor will tell you which to use. The choice of printer or file is selected
from the Print Dialog window.

Step 20

Position your mouse pointer over the menu item Select at the top of the screen and click
your mouse button. A list of the Select menu functions (shown in Figure 4-15) will appear.

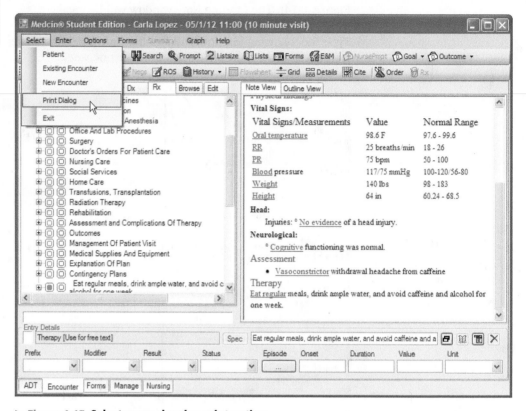

▶ Figure 4-15 **Select menu showing print option.**

Move the mouse pointer vertically down the list until Print Dialog is highlighted and
then click the mouse button. The Print Data window will be invoked.

The two panes on the left list items that are available for printing. A check box is used
to indicate which items you wish to print. If the box next to "Current Encounter" does
not have a check mark, position your mouse pointer over it and click the mouse button.
A check mark should appear in the box (see Figure 4-16).

The right pane displays a preview of what is to be printed.

Located below the right pane are two rows of buttons. Those of interest to us are
as follows:

Print and Close   Prints the items selected with check marks to a local or
networked printer. This produces a paper copy you can
hand in to your instructor.

Export to XPS File   Outputs the items selected with check marks to a file on
your local computer. The file can be copied to a disk or
flash drive or e-mailed to your instructor. The XPS file is
a Microsoft file that can be viewed with Internet Explorer.

► **Figure 4-16 Print Data window.**

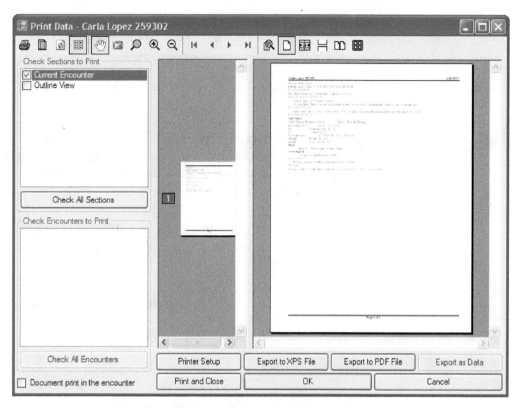

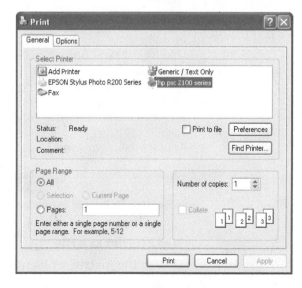

Export to PDF File   Outputs the items selected with check marks to a file on your local computer. The file can be copied to a disk or flash drive or e-mailed to your instructor. The PDF file is a file that can be viewed with Adobe Acrobat Reader®.

Your instructor will tell you which method is appropriate for your class.

Step 21: Print a Paper Copy of the Encounter Note

If the instructor wants you to export a file, skip this step and proceed to Step 22.

If the instructor wants you to print out a paper copy, locate the button labeled "Print and Close" and click the mouse.

Depending on how your computer is set up, an additional print window from the operating system may appear. Figure 4-17 shows an example. Yours may

► **Figure 4-17 Additional Print window from operating system.**

be different, but if you see a printer dialog similar to this, verify that the printer name is the printer you want to use and then click your mouse on the button labeled "Print."

If you need assistance printing, ask your instructor.

Alert

Some printers may close the print window before the printing has even started. Therefore, do not exit the Student Edition program or go on to another exercise until you have your printout in hand. You could lose your work.

Compare your printout to Figure 4-18 and then give it to your instructor. You may print extra copies by repeating steps 20 and 21 before exiting the Student Edition software.

Carla Lopez   Page 1 of 1

Student: *your name or ID here*
Patient: Carla Lopez: F: 12/30/1984: 5/01/2012 11:00 AM
Chief complaint
The Chief Complaint is: Headaches for more than 5 days.
History of present illness
 Carla Lopez is a 27 year old female.
 She reported: Chronic/recurring headaches recently worse which is inadequately controlled and occurring daily.
Personal history
Behavioral: Daily coffee consumption was 7-8 cups per day has recently decreased because she stopped all coffee.
Physical findings
Vital Signs:

Vital Signs/Measurements	Value	Normal Range
Oral temperature	98.6 F	(97.6 - 99.6)
RR	25 breaths/min	(18 - 26)
PR	75 bpm	(50 - 100)
Blood pressure	117/75 mmHg	(100-120/56-80)
Weight	140 lbs	(98 - 183)
Height	64 in	(60.24 - 68.5)

Head:
 Injuries: ° No evidence of a head injury.
Neurological:
 ° Cognitive functioning was normal.
Assessment
 • Vasoconstrictor withdrawal headache from caffeine
Therapy
Eat Regular meals, drink ample water, and avoid caffeine and alcohol for one week.

▶ Figure 4-18 **Printed encounter note for Carla Lopez.**

Step 22: Print to a File

Unless the instructor wants you to export to a file, omit this step.

To export to a file instead of printing to paper, click the mouse pointer on the appropriate button (either "Export to XPS File" or "Export to PDF File" as directed by your instructor).

The action of either button is to create a file on your computer in the directory named "My Documents." The file name will include the student name or ID you entered when you logged in plus the date and time. The file name ends in either "XPS" or "PDF."

When the file has been successfully created, a confirmation similar to Figure 4-19 will be displayed.

▶ Figure 4-19 **Export to File confirmation.**

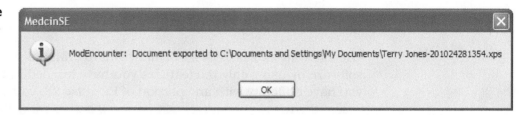

Write down the file name shown in the dialog box, then click on the OK button.

Once the file has been created, you can copy it to a disk or e-mail it, as directed by your instructor. Use the computer operating system to locate the file on your computer. It will be located in the directory named "My Documents." Follow your instructor's directions for handing in your file.

The instructor can view or print the student XPS file using Internet Explorer as shown in Figure 4-20. The instructor can view or print the student PDF file using Adobe Acrobat Reader (not shown.)

▶ Figure 4-20 **Student XPS file displayed using Internet Explorer.**

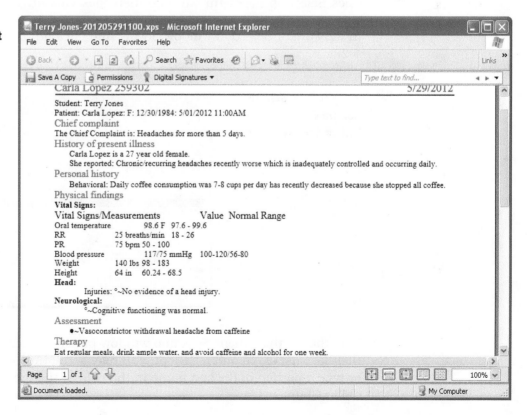

Invoking the Print Dialog Window from the Toolbar Another way to invoke the Print Dialog window is by clicking the button labeled "Print" on the Toolbar at the top of your screen (highlighted orange and circled in red in Figure 4-21). You can print out or export copies of the encounter note as frequently as you like and at anytime during an exercise.

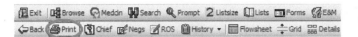

▶ Figure 4-21 **Print Button on Toolbar (circled in red).**

Documenting Brief Patient Visits

The following two exercises will allow you to evaluate your knowledge of the software by using only the features you have learned in Chapters 3 and 4. If you have difficulty with any portion of Exercise 28, you should review and repeat the relevant exercises in Chapter 3 before doing Exercise 29.

Guided Exercise 28: Documenting a Visit for a Common Cold

Patient Howard Cook feels like he has caught some sort of "bug." Like many patients who have a cold, he wants to see his doctor, so the medical office has scheduled an office visit for him. Using what you have learned so far, document Mr. Cook's brief exam.

Step 1

If you have not already done so, start the Student Edition software.

Click Select on the Menu bar, and then click Patient.

In the Patient Selection window, locate and click on "Howard Cook" (see Figure 4-22).

▶ Figure 4-22 **Selecting Howard Cook from the Patient Selection window.**

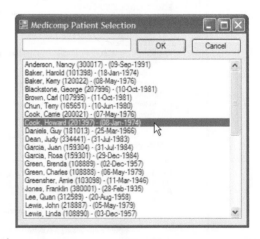

Note that in the Patient Selection window patients are listed alphabetically by their last name. To find a patient, you may scroll the list to locate the patient, or type a portion of the last name in the field at the top of the window as you did in Chapter 3.

Step 2

Click Select on the Menu bar, and then click New Encounter.

Scroll the drop-down list to locate the reason "Office Visit," as shown in Figure 4-23, and then click on it.

You may use the current date for this exercise, but be certain that you have selected the correct reason before clicking on the OK button.

▶ Figure 4-23 **New encounter for an "Office Visit."**

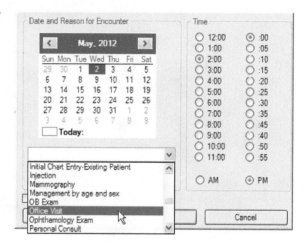

Step 3

Enter the chief complaint by locating the button in the Toolbar labeled "Chief" and clicking on it.

In the dialog window that opens, type **Patient reported cold or flu.**

Compare your screen to Figure 4-24 before clicking on the button labeled "Close the note form."

▶ Figure 4-24 **Chief complaint: Patient reported cold or flu.**

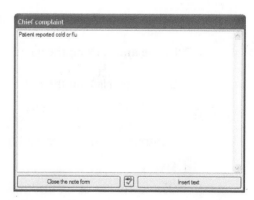

Step 4

The patient reports a headache, runny nose, and sneezing. Enter the patient's symptoms using the list of findings on the Sx tab.

Expand the tree of Medcin findings.

Locate and click on the small plus sign next to "head-related symptoms."

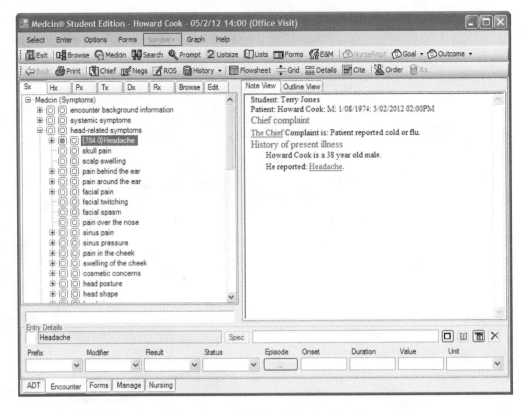

▶ Figure 4-25 Symptom: headache.

Locate and click on the red button next to the following finding:

- (red button) Headache

Compare your screen to Figure 4-25.

Step 5

Scroll the list of Sx findings downward to locate "otolaryngeal symptoms." Expand the tree of findings further:

Click on the small plus sign next to "otolaryngeal symptoms."

Locate and click on the small plus sign next to "nose."

Locate and click on the small plus sign next to "nasal discharge."

Locate and click on the red button for the following finding:

- (red button) Watery

Compare your screen to Figure 4-26.

Step 6

Scroll the list of Sx findings further downward to locate and click on the red button for the following finding:

- (red button) Sneezing

Compare your screen to Figure 4-27.

Step 7

The patient does not smoke. Enter this fact in the patient's history:

Click on the Hx tab.

► Figure 4-26 **Symptom: watery nasal discharge.**

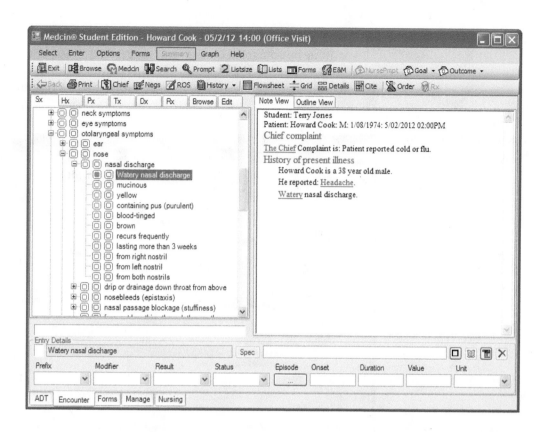

► Figure 4-27 **Symptom: Sneezing.**

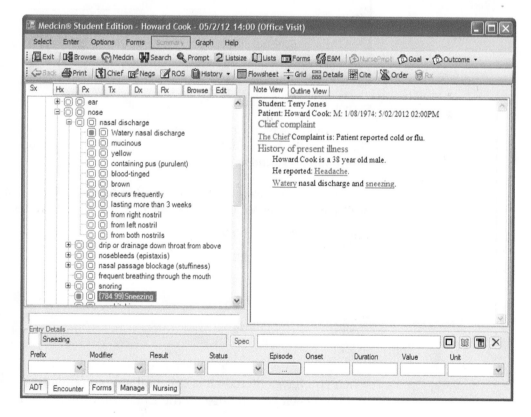

Expand the tree of Medcin findings.

Locate and click on the small plus sign next to "social history."

Locate and click on the small plus sign next to "behavioral history."

Locate and click on the blue button next to the following finding:

- (blue button) tobacco use

The description will change to "No Tobacco Use." Compare your screen to Figure 4-28.

▶ Figure 4-28 History: No tobacco use.

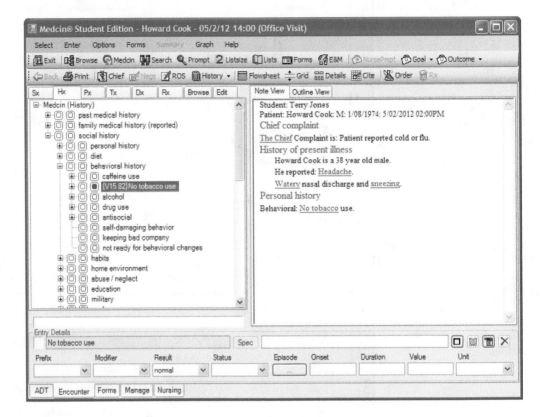

Step 8

Locate and click on the button labeled "Forms" in the top row of buttons on the Toolbar. The tabs at the bottom of the screen will automatically change to the Forms tab. The Forms Manager window will be invoked.

Locate and double-click on the form labeled "Vitals." The form shown in Figure 4-29 will be displayed. Enter Mr. Cook's vital signs in the corresponding fields as follows:

Temperature:	**99.7**
Respiration:	**25**
Pulse:	**65**
BP:	**120/80**
Height:	**72**
Weight:	**175**

When you have entered all of the vital signs, compare your screen to Figure 4-29 and then click your mouse on the Encounter tab at the bottom of the screen.

Step 9

The clinician examines the patient's head, eyes, ears, nose, inside of mouth, and lungs.

Begin recording information obtained from the physical exam by clicking on the Px tab.

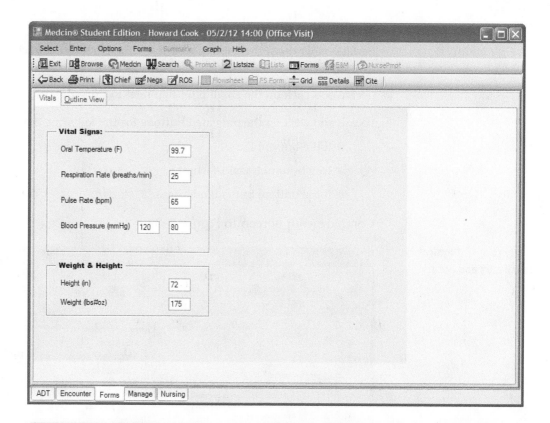

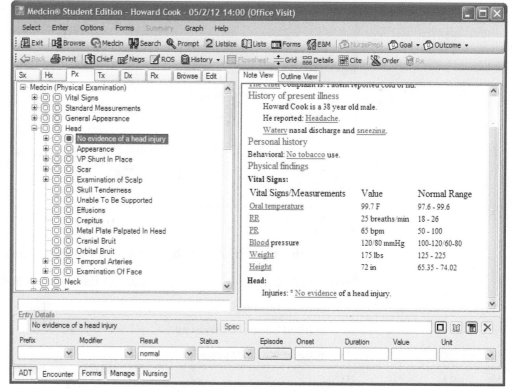

Locate and click on the small plus sign next to "Head."

Locate and click on the blue button next to the following finding:

● (blue button) Exam for Evidence of injury

The description will change to "No evidence of a head injury." Compare your screen to Figure 4-30.

Step 10

Scroll further down the list of physical findings to locate and click on the small plus sign next to "Ears, Nose, Throat."

Locate and click on the small plus sign next to "Nose."

Locate and click on the indicated buttons for the following findings:

- (blue button) Ears
- (red button) Nasal Discharge
- (blue button) Sinus tenderness

Compare your screen to Figure 4-31.

▶ Figure 4-31 **Physical exam: ears and nose.**

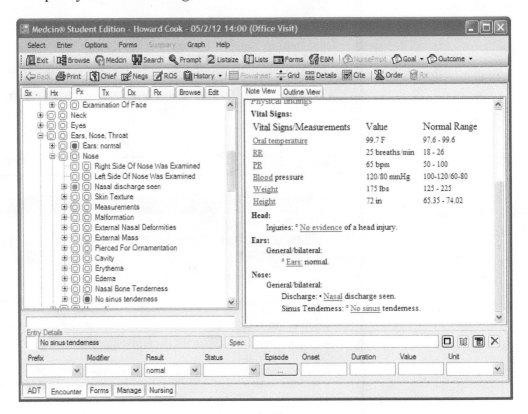

Step 11

Scroll further down the list of physical findings to locate "Lungs."

Locate and click on the indicated buttons for the following findings:

- (blue button) Upper Airway
- (blue button) Oral cavity
- (blue button) Lungs

Compare your screen to Figure 4-32.

Step 12

The clinician concludes the patient has a common cold, and tells him to rest and drink plenty of fluids. Record the assessment by clicking on the Dx tab:

Expand the tree of findings.

Locate and click on the small plus sign next to "ENT Disorders."

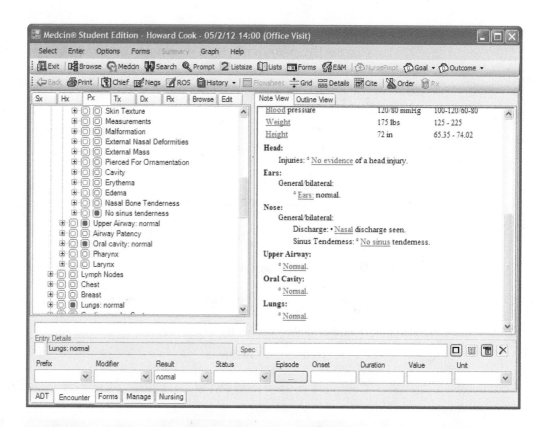

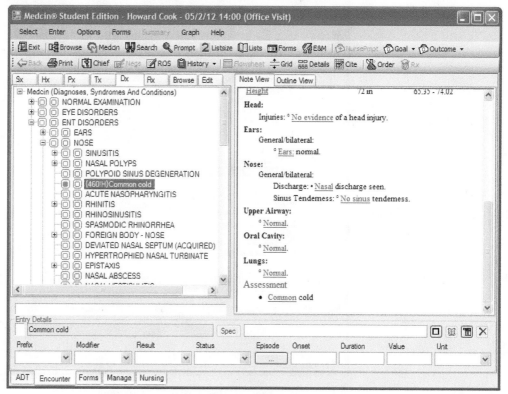

Locate and click on the small plus sign next to "Nose."

Locate and click on the following finding:

- (red button) Common cold

Compare your screen to Figure 4-33.

Step 13

Record the plan by clicking on the Rx tab. Expand the tree of findings:

Locate and click on the small plus sign next to "Basic Management Procedures and Services."

Scroll the list downward until you locate "Nutrition and Hydration Services," then click on the small plus sign next to it.

Locate and click on the following finding:

- (red button) Fluids

Expand the tree of findings further:

Locate and click on the small plus sign next to "Education and Instructions."

Locate and click on the small plus sign next to Instructions for Patient.

Locate and click on the following finding:

- (red button) Bed rest

Compare your screen to Figure 4-34.

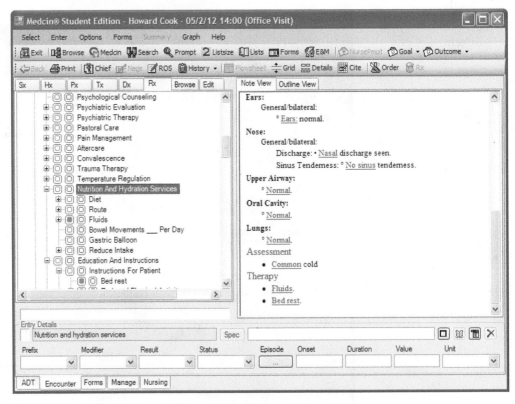

▶ Figure 4-34 **Therapy plan: patient instructions.**

Step 14

Print your completed encounter note:

Click on the Print button on the Toolbar at the top of your screen to invoke the Print Data window.

Look at the upper left pane of the window. If the box next to "Current Encounter" does not have a check mark, position your mouse pointer over it and click the mouse button. A check mark should appear in the box.

Click on either the button labeled "Print and Close" or "Export to XPS File" or "Export to PDF File" as directed by your instructor.

Compare your printout or exported file to Figure 4-35. If it is correct, hand it in to your instructor. If there are any differences (other than the date and patient age), review the previous steps in the exercise and find your error.

Howard Cook   Page 1 of 1

Student: *your name or ID here*
Patient: Howard Cook: M: 1/08/1974: 5/02/2012 02:00 PM
Chief complaint
The Chief Complaint is: Patient reported cold or flu.
History of present illness
     Howard Cook is a 38 year old male.
     He reported: Headache.
     Watery nasal discharge and sneezing.
Personal history
Behavioral: No tobacco use.
Physical findings
Vital Signs:

Vital Signs/Measurements	Value	Normal Range
Oral temperature	99.7 F	97.6 - 99.6
RR	25 breaths/min	18 - 26
PR	65 bpm	50 - 100
Blood pressure	120/80 mmHg	100-120/60-80
Weight	175 lbs	125 - 225
Height	72 in	65.35 - 74.02

Head:
     Injuries: ° No evidence of a head injury.
Ears:
     General/bilateral:
      ° Ears: normal.
Nose:
     General/bilateral:
      Discharge: • Nasal discharge seen.
      Sinus Tenderness: ° No sinus tenderness.
Upper Airway:
     ° Normal.
Oral Cavity:
     ° Normal.
Lungs:
     ° Normal.
Assessment
     • Common cold
Therapy
     • Fluids.
     • Bed rest.

▶ Figure 4-35 **Printed encounter note for Howard Cook.**

Once you have successfully completed this exercise, you should be comfortable with the general process of locating findings and expanding the tree to view additional findings. Future exercises in this book will instruct you to expand the tree so that it lists multiple findings by clicking on several small plus signs in one step.

Critical Thinking Exercise 29: A Patient with Sinusitis

This exercise will help you evaluate how well you can use the Student Edition software to create an encounter note. The exercise provides step-by-step instructions, but does not provide screen figures for reference. The exercises in Chapter 3 covered each feature used in this exercise. If you have difficulty at any step during this exercise, refer to the Chapter 3 Summary where a table lists each feature and the corresponding exercise for that feature.

Patient John Lewis has been experiencing stuffy sinus pain. The medical office has scheduled a brief office visit for him to see the nurse practitioner. Using what you have learned so far, document Mr. Lewis's brief exam.

Step 1

If you have not already done so, start the Student Edition software.

Click Select on the Menu bar, and then click Patient.

In the Patient Selection window, locate and click on "John Lewis."

Step 2

Click Select on the Menu bar, and then click New Encounter.

Select the reason "10 minute visit" from the drop-down list.

Make sure you have selected the reason correctly. You may use the current date for this exercise.

Step 3

Enter the chief complaint by locating the button in the Toolbar labeled "Chief" and clicking on it.

In the dialog window that opens, type **Stuffy sinus**.

Click on the button labeled "Close the note form."

Step 4

The patient reports a sinus pain, stuffy nose, and nasal discharge. Enter the patient's symptoms using the list of findings on the Sx tab:

Expand the tree of Medcin findings by locating and clicking on the small plus sign next to "head-related symptoms."

Locate and click on the indicated button for following finding:

- (red button) Sinus pain

Step 5

Scroll the list of Sx findings downward to locate "otolaryngeal symptoms."

Expand the tree of Sx findings by locating and clicking on the small plus sign next to each of the following:

> otolaryngeal symptoms

> nose

Locate and click on the indicated button for the following findings:
- (red button) Nasal Discharge
- (red button) Nasal passage blockage (stuffiness)

Step 6

The patient reports smoking for 20 years. Enter this fact in the patient's history:

Click on the Hx tab.

Expand the tree of Hx findings by locating and clicking on the small plus sign next to each of the following:

> social history

> behavioral history

> tobacco use

Locate and click on the indicated button for the following finding:
- (red button) current smoker

Step 7

Locate the Value field in the Entry Details section at the bottom of the screen.

Type 20 in the field and press the enter key.

The description will change to "Current smoker was 20 years."

Step 8

Locate and click on the button labeled "Forms" on the Toolbar to invoke the Forms Manager window. Locate and double-click on the form labeled "Vitals."

Enter Mr. Lewis's vital signs in the corresponding fields as follows:

Temperature:	**96.7**
Respiration:	**27**
Pulse:	**67**
BP:	**120/87**
Height:	**68**
Weight:	**177**

When you have entered all of the vital signs, click your mouse on the Encounter tab at the bottom of the screen.

Step 9

The clinician examines the patient's head, eyes, ears, nose, inside of mouth, and lungs.

Begin recording information obtained from the physical exam by clicking on the Px tab.

Locate and click on the small plus sign next to "Head."

Locate and click on the indicated button for the following finding:

- (blue button) Exam for Evidence of injury

The description will change to "No evidence of a head injury."

Step 10

Scroll the list of Physical findings downward to locate "Eyes."

Locate and click on the indicated button for the following finding:

- (blue button) Eyes

Expand the tree of Px findings by locating and clicking on the small plus sign next to each of the following:

Ears, Nose, Throat

Nose

Nasal Discharge

Locate and click on the indicated buttons for the following findings:

- (blue button) Ears
- (red button) Nasal Discharge
- (red button) Sinus tenderness
- (blue button) Oral cavity
- (blue button) Pharynx

Step 11

Scroll the list of Px findings further downward to locate and click on the small plus sign next to Lungs.

Locate and click on the blue button for the following finding:

- (blue button) Percussion

Step 12

The clinician concludes the patient has acute sinusitis that is already improving. Record the assessment by clicking on the Dx tab:

Expand the tree of Dx findings by locating and clicking on the small plus sign next to each of the following:

ENT Disorders

Nose

Sinusitis

Locate and click on the red button for the following finding:

- Acute

Step 13

Locate the Status field in the Entry Details section at the bottom of the screen. Click your mouse on the button with the down arrow in the field. A drop-down list of choices will appear.

Locate and click on the status "improving."

The assessment will change to read "Acute sinusitis which is improving."

Step 14

The clinician advises Mr. Lewis to continue taking over-the-counter antihistamines, drink plenty of fluids, and quit smoking. Record the plan by clicking on the Rx tab:

Locate and click on the small plus sign next to "Basic Management Procedures and Services."

Scroll the list downward until you locate "Nutrition and Hydration Services," then click on the small plus sign next to it.

Locate and click on the indicated button for the following finding:

- (red button) Fluids

Scroll down the list until you locate "Education and Instructions," then click on the small plus sign next to it.

Locate and click on the small plus sign next to "Instructions for Patient."

Locate and click on the indicated button for the following finding:

- (red button) Abstinence from smoking

Scroll the list downward until you locate "Medications and Vaccines," then click on the small plus sign next to it.

Locate and highlight the medicine "Antihistamines," but do not click the red or blue button.

Locate the Prefix field in the Entry Details section at the bottom of the screen. Click your mouse on the button with the down arrow in the field. A drop-down list of choices will appear.

Locate and click on the status "continue."

Locate the free-text field in the Entry Details section at the bottom of the screen. (It is located just above the button labeled "Episode.")

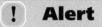

! Alert

Do not close or exit the encounter until you have a printed copy in your hand. You will lose your work if you exit before printing.

Type **OTC** in the field and press the enter key. "OTC" means over-the-counter.

The description should now read "Continue antihistamines OTC."

Step 15

Print your completed encounter note:

Click on the Print button on the Toolbar at the top of your screen to invoke the Print Data window.

Be certain there is a check mark in the box next to "Current Encounter" and then click on either the appropriate button to print or export a file, as directed by your instructor.

Compare your printout or exported file to Figure 4-36. If it is correct, hand it in to your instructor. If there are any differences (other than the date and patient age), review the previous steps in the exercise and find your error.

Student: *your name or ID here*
Patient: John Lewis: M: 5/05/1979: 5/03/2012 02:15 PM
Chief complaint
The Chief Complaint is: Stuffy sinus.
History of present illness
      John Lewis is a 32 year old male.
      He reported: Sinus pain.
      Nasal discharge and nasal passage blockage.
Personal history
Behavioral: Current Smoker was 20 years.
Physical findings
Vital Signs:

Vital Signs/Measurements	Value	Normal Range
Oral temperature	96.7 F	97.6 - 99.6
RR	27 breaths/min	18 - 26
PR	67 bpm	50 - 100
Blood pressure	120/87 mmHg	100-120/60-80
Weight	177 lbs	125 - 225
Height	68 in	65.35 - 74.02

Head:
      Injuries: ° No evidence of a head injury.
Eyes:
      General/bilateral:
          ° Eyes: normal.
Ears:
      General/bilateral:
          ° Ears: normal.
Nose:
      General/bilateral:
          Discharge: • Nasal discharge seen.
          Sinus Tenderness: • Tenderness of sinuses.
Oral Cavity:
      ° Normal.
Pharynx:
      ° Normal.
Lungs:
      ° Chest was normal to percussion.
Assessment
      • Acute sinusitis which is improving
Therapy
      • Fluids.
      • Continue antihistamines OTC.
Counseling/Education
      • Abstinence from smoking

▶ Figure 4-36 **Printed encounter note for John Lewis.**

Chapter Four Summary

In this chapter you have performed exercises intended to increase your familiarity with the Student Edition software and thereby increase your speed of data entry. You have also learned how to print out encounter notes or export them as files. You can print the encounter note at any time and as often as you like while practicing your exercises. However, remember not to quit or exit the program **until you are sure the encounter note has printed**. Once you exit, you will lose your work.

As you continue through the course you can refer to the Exercise 27 in this chapter if you need to remember how to print or export a file. You can also repeat any of the exercises in this chapter to increase your skills using the software. You should not proceed with the remainder of the text until you can perform the exercises in this chapter with ease.

Testing Your Knowledge of Chapter 4

1. Why is it important to print your work before exiting?
2. What does the Export to PDF File button do?
3. How many cups of coffee per day had Carla Lopez been drinking before she quit?
4. What Entry Details field was used to record that Carla's headaches were inadequately controlled?
5. How long had she had her condition?
6. How long was John Lewis's office visit scheduled for?
7. Which of Howard Cook's symptoms did you record under the "otolaryngeal symptoms" finding?
8. Does Howard smoke?
9. Did Howard report sinus pain or tenderness?
10. What was the doctor's assessment (diagnosis) of Howard Cook's condition?
11. What was the doctor's plan (Rx) for Howard Cook?
12. What was John Lewis's chief complaint?
13. On what tab did you record that John Lewis smoked?
14. What does the acronym OTC stand for?
15. You should have produced encounter note documents for three patients, which you printed or exported to files. If you have not already done so, hand these in to your instructor with this test. The encounter notes will count as a portion of your grade.

5

Learning to Use Search and Prompt

Learning Outcomes

After completing this chapter, you should be able to:

- Use the Student Edition Toolbar
- Search for a finding using the Search button
- Understand and use the Prompt feature
- Understand and use the List Size feature
- Record orders for tests
- Record orders for an x-ray

Tools That Speed Data Entry

Earlier, it was stated that the goal of many EHR systems is to document the visit completely before the patient ever leaves the office. To document in real time, you must be able to quickly navigate and enter findings. To aid the healthcare professional in this goal, an EHR needs to present the finding the user needs when it is needed.

In this chapter, you will learn about additional features that help a healthcare professional enter data more quickly. These include using the Toolbar and the Search and Prompt features, which are invoked from the Toolbar. The next two chapters will discuss Lists and Forms, both of which are also invoked from the Toolbar.

Encounter Tab Toolbar

Located at the top of your screen are two rows of icon buttons called a "Toolbar." In previous exercises you have already used several of the buttons on the Toolbar. As you practice the remaining exercises in this book, you will learn about and use additional buttons on the Toolbar.

You may have noticed that different buttons appear on the Toolbar when you switch to the Forms tab. Toolbar buttons also change when you access the Management tab. These variations in the Toolbar on other tabs will be covered as they occur. For now, we will focus on the Toolbar as it appears when you use the Encounter tab (see Figure 5-1).

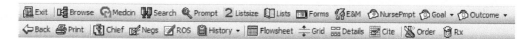

▶ Figure 5-1 **Toolbar as it appears on the Encounter tab.**

A quick reference guide to the buttons available on the Toolbar when you are on the Encounter tab is provided here. You will learn more about the buttons by using them in the exercises. You can refer back to this guide any time you are unsure of the function of a button on the Toolbar.

Top Row:

Exit	Exits the Student Edition program and closes the window.
Browse	Displays the current finding's position in the Medcin nomenclature hierarchy using a separate tab.
Medcin	Displays the Medcin nomenclature in the data entry trees.
Search	Invokes the Search dialog window.
Prompt	Dynamically generates a list based on the finding currently highlighted.
Listsize	Increases or decreases the number of findings displayed from a list.
Lists	Invokes the Lists Manager window.
Forms	Invokes the Forms Manager window.
E&M	Calculates the CPT-4 Evaluation and Management (billing) code based on the findings recorded in the encounter note.

The **NursePmpt** (Nurse Prompt), **Goal**, and **Outcome** buttons are not used for exercises in this book.

Bottom Row:

Back	This is used to re-invoke the previous entry mode selection.
Print	Invokes the Print Data dialog window.
Chief	Invokes a finding note window specifically for the patient's chief complaint.
Negs	Automatically selects "normal" for all findings in the Sx or Px tab that are not already selected. In most cases this is the blue button.
ROS	Review of Systems; can be on or off. When on (button changes color) all symptoms selected are grouped in the Review of Systems category. When off, symptoms selected are grouped in the History of Present Illness category.
History	Automatically sets the prefix of the current finding to "History of."
Order	Automatically sets the prefix of a current finding in the Tx or Rx tab to "Ordered."
Rx	Invokes the Prescription Writer window for medications in the Rx tab.

The **Flowsheet, Grid, Details**, and **Cite** buttons are not used for exercises in this book.

Using buttons on the Toolbar speeds up data entry by invoking windows when convenient and by reducing the number of items a clinician must click to complete a note.

Search and Prompt Features

The exercises so far have used relatively simple exams with findings that were fairly easy to locate. Actual patient encounters, however, often involve multiple problems, and more complex exams require more time to document. Is there a faster way to find what you are looking for than just scrolling the navigation list and expanding the trees? Yes!

As you learned in Chapter 3, the Medcin nomenclature has hundreds of thousands of findings. The challenges with large clinical vocabularies include:

◆ How can you locate a finding among hundreds of thousands?

◆ Does the nomenclature use the same term for the finding as you do?

◆ Where are other related findings?

The Search feature provides a quick way for the healthcare professional to locate a desired finding in the nomenclature. Search produces a list of the findings almost instantly. Medcin addresses semantic differences in medical terms in several ways:

1. Search performs automatic word completion so if you search for *knee* but the finding is for *knees*, the system will still find it.

2. Medcin includes an extensive list of synonyms that are used in an alternate word search. For example, if you search for *knee injury*, the search results will also include findings for *knee burns, knee trauma,* and *fractured patella,* among others.

3. Search identifies related findings in other tabs so that when you search for a word or phrase in a particular tab, related findings are automatically available in the other tabs. This means that when you are using search while documenting a patient exam, as you proceed through the exam, the other tabs may already have related findings that you will need.

How Search Works

Search is not designed to find every instance that contains the words being searched because the search results would often have too many findings. Instead, search uses the Medcin hierarchy (the tree view you have expanded in previous exercises). It finds and shows the highest level match and does not list all of the expanded findings below it.

For example, in Chapter 3 you did an exercise with a "Headache" finding during which you expanded the tree to show many types of headache. If you searched for *headache*, the search results would display the finding "Headache" with a small plus sign next to it. If you wanted to peruse the various types of headaches, you would click on the plus sign to expand the tree. However, if you search for *migraine headache*, the search results will show "Headache" with the tree already expanded to the "migraine" finding.

The Search feature always begins its search in the tab you are currently in when you start the search. If applicable search results are found in another tab but none in the current tab, the software will automatically change to the first tab with results. The order of the tabs you see on the screen is the same order in which search will display the results. For example, if you are on the Tx tab when you search and there are no results for Tx, but there are results for the Dx tab, it will automatically change the nomenclature pane to the Dx tab because that is the next tab in sequence.

The next two exercises will give you experience using three new features. Do not begin Exercise 30 unless there is enough class time remaining to complete both Exercises 30 and 31.

Guided Exercise 30: Using Search and Prompt

Although this exercise does not produce a very thorough encounter note, it will teach you how to use the Search and Prompt features as well as several other buttons on the Toolbar.

The patient, Paul Mitsuhiro, has been referred to the physician with suspected angina. The doctor ascertains that the patient is not in any immediate danger and is therefore going to schedule a complete workup later this week. In the meantime, the doctor wants to order some tests so that the results will be ready when the patient returns for his more complete exam. A medical assistant is going to enter the chief complaint and vital signs and record the doctor's orders.

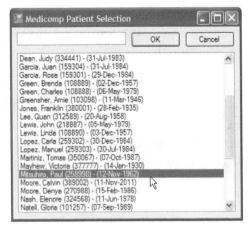

▶ Figure 5-2 **Selecting Paul Mitsuhiro from the Patient Selection window.**

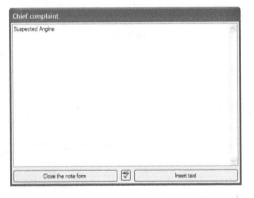

▶ Figure 5-3 **Chief complaint window for suspected angina.**

To quickly locate the desired findings, you can start with a known symptom or disease and work forward, rather than navigate the entire Medcin nomenclature of findings. We will use the Search function to do this.

Step 1

If you have not already done so, start the Student Edition software.

Click Select on the Menu bar, and then click Patient.

In the Patient Selection window, locate and click on "Paul Mitsuhiro" as shown in Figure 5-2.

Step 2

Click Select on the Menu bar, and then click New Encounter.

You may use the current date and time for this exercise.

Select the reason "Office Visit" from the drop-down Reason list. Click on the OK button.

In the next two steps, the medical assistant enters the chief complaint and vital signs.

Step 3

Enter the chief complaint by locating the button in the Toolbar labeled "Chief" and clicking on it.

In the dialog window that opens, type **Suspected Angina**.

Compare your screen to Figure 5-3 before clicking on the button labeled "Close the note form."

Step 4

Enter Mr. Mitsuhiro's vital signs using the Vitals form located on the Forms tab (as you have done in the previous exercises):

Locate and click on the button labeled Forms in the Toolbar at the top of your screen. (If you have difficulty locating the Forms tab or Forms button, refer to Chapter 4, Figure 4-9.)

Select the form labeled "Vitals" from the list in the Forms Manager window.

Enter Paul Mitsuhiro's vital signs in the corresponding fields as follows:

Temperature:	**98.6**
Respiration:	**22**
Pulse:	**70**
BP:	**130/85**
Height:	**65**
Weight:	**138**

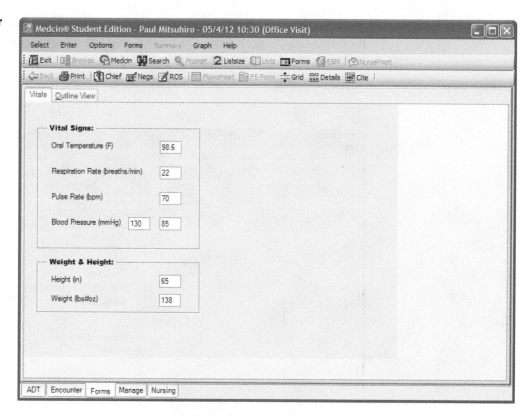

When you have finished, compare your screen to Figure 5-4. If it is correct,
click on the tab labeled Encounter at the bottom of the window.

Step 5

Locate the Search button on the Toolbar near the top of the screen. The Search
icon resembles a small pair of binoculars. It is highlighted orange in Figure 5-5.

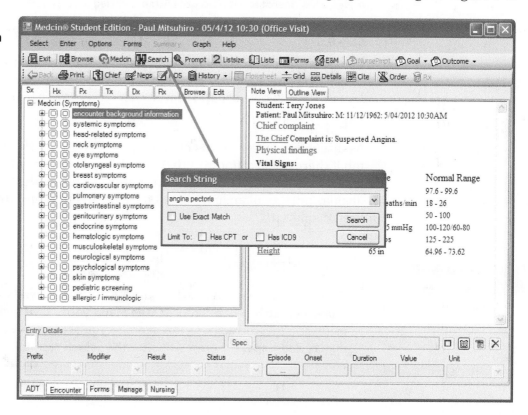

Click your mouse on it to invoke the Search String window. Position your mouse in the Search String field and enter the medical term **angina pectoris**. Verify that you have spelled this correctly, then click the button in the box labeled "Search."

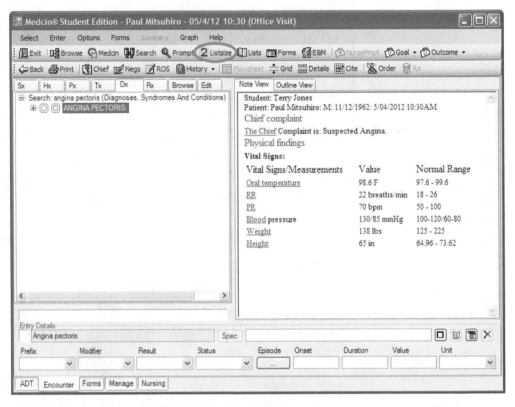

▶ Figure 5-6 **Search results (Listsize button is circled in red.)**

Step 6

Compare your screen to Figure 5-6, which shows that search has succeeded. Notice that you started the search on the Sx tab but the screen is now on the Dx tab. This is because the search was for a very specific pair of words that did not exist in the other tabs.

As discussed earlier in this chapter, the Search result displays in the current tab if there are any findings that match the search string; otherwise, it displays in the first tab with findings that match. Had the search simply been for angina, "history of angina" would have been found and the Hx tab would have been displayed.

Note

No Results?

If your screen does not match Figure 5-6 or you received the message "nothing found to match search," repeat step 5 and verify that you have spelled the medical terms correctly. In this exercise you are searching for a very specific match, and a spelling error will alter the search results.

Step 7

Locate the button labeled "Listsize" on the Toolbar near the top of the screen. The List Size icon is a teal square with a black numeral (from 1 to 3) in it. It is circled in red in Figure 5-6. As the name implies, the List Size feature controls the number of findings that will be displayed in a "prompt list."

Each time you click the mouse on the Listsize button, it changes to the next number in sequence, from 1 to 3. When it reaches 3, it will start again at 1 the next time the button is clicked. You will see how List Size affects the nomenclature pane in step 9.

For this step, set the list size to **1**. If the list size is currently greater than 1, click your mouse over the icon repeatedly until it displays a "1."

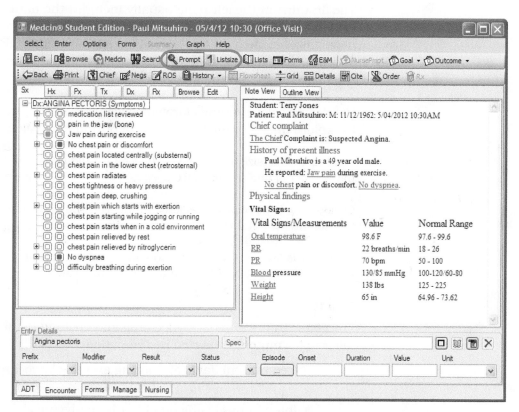

▶ Figure 5-7 **Sx tab displaying findings related to angina (shown after findings selected).**

Step 8

Locate the Prompt button on the Toolbar near the top of the screen. The Prompt icon resembles a small magnifying glass. It is circled in red in Figure 5-7. The full name of the feature is "Prompt with current finding." This feature generates a list of findings that are clinically related to the finding currently highlighted. For this step, angina pectoris should be highlighted in blue on your screen.

Click your mouse on the Prompt button at this time.

Once the list is displayed, you can use it just like you have been using the full nomenclature in previous exercises. That is, you can expand the tree of displayed findings by clicking the small plus signs. You can record findings by clicking on the red or blue buttons next to the findings. You also can change tabs; however, the findings displayed in the other tabs will be limited to those that are clinically related to the finding that was highlighted when you clicked the Prompt button.

Step 9

The left pane should have automatically changed to the Sx tab; if it did not, click on the tab labeled Sx.

Compare the list in the left pane of your screen to Figure 5-7, ignoring the red and blue buttons for the moment. Note that the list of findings is much shorter than is normally displayed in the Sx tab.

The first line in the left pane usually includes the name or source of the list. Heretofore, this was just the name of the tab, for example, Medcin (Symptoms); now, however, the first line reads "Dx: ANGINA PECTORIS (Symptoms)." This indicates that the list is limited to findings that are clinically related to the diagnosis angina pectoris.

Before you select findings for your encounter note, this is a good opportunity to explore the function of the Listsize button discussed in step 7:

Click on the Listsize button once. The icon should change to the numeral 2; note that the number of findings has increased.

Click on the Listsize button again and the icon should change to the numeral 3; note that the number of findings has increased even more.

Click on the Listsize button one more time and the icon should change back to a 1 and the list of findings should return to the shortest list.

Step 10

Proceed with the exercise by locating and clicking the indicated button for the following symptoms reported by the patient:

- (red button) Jaw pain during exercise (myocardial)
- (blue button) Chest pain or discomfort
- (blue button) Difficulty breathing (dyspnea)

Compare your screen to the selected red and blue buttons in Figure 5-7.

Step 11

The patient does not smoke, and denies any history of high blood pressure or diabetes. Click on the Hx tab and enter the patient's history information by locating and clicking on the indicated buttons for the following history findings:

- (blue button) current smoker
- (blue button) history of hypertension (Systemic)
- (blue button) history of diabetes mellitus

Compare your screen to Figure 5-8 before proceeding.

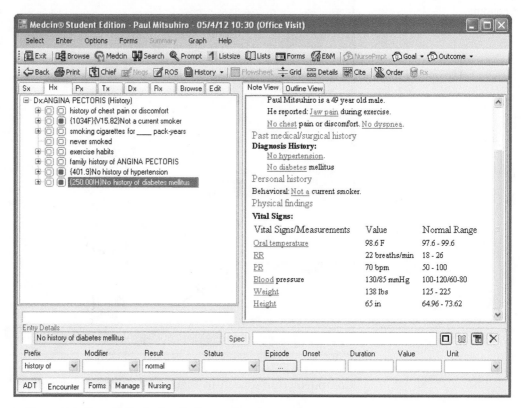

▶ Figure 5-8 **Hx tab displaying findings related to angina.**

Step 12

Today's visit is preliminary and mainly to order and perform some tests before a complete exam scheduled later in the week. However, a brief physical is performed by the clinician.

Click on the Listsize button until the list size is **2**.

Click on the Px tab. Notice that two findings are already selected; these are vital signs entered earlier.

Enter the physical exam information by locating and clicking on the following findings:

- (blue button) Pulse Rhythm Irregular
- (blue button) Hypotension
- (blue button) Bradycardia (by Auscultation)
- (blue button) Heart Sounds S3
- (blue button) Heart Sounds S4
- (blue button) Heart Sounds Gallop
- (blue button) Abdomen Tenderness Direct
- (blue button) Pallor Generalized

► Figure 5-9 **Px tab: physical exam findings related
to angina.**

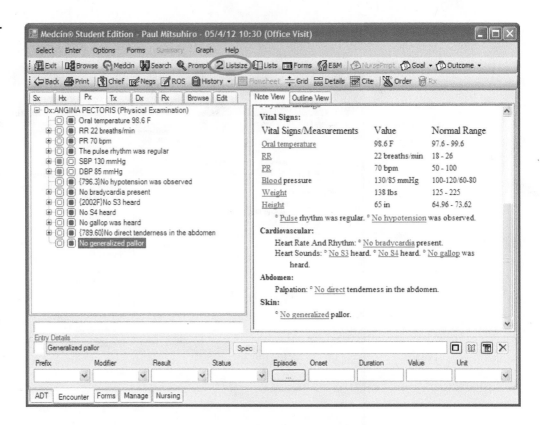

Compare your screen to Figure 5-9 before proceeding.

Do not exit the program until you have completed the following exercise.

Guided Exercise 31: Ordering Diagnostic Tests

Continuing with Mr. Mitsuhiro's visit, this exercise will explore several methods
of recording tests and orders.

Step 13

Click on the Listsize button until it displays the numeral **1**.

Click on the Tx tab, which will display a list of tests that might be ordered for angina
pectoris.

When a test is performed at the medical facility, the fact is documented by clicking on
the red button next to the test name. Locate and click on the following finding:

    ● (red button) Electrocardiogram

The encounter note should now read "An ECG was performed," as shown in
Figure 5-10.

Step 14

Although some tests, such as electrocardiograms, are performed in the office,
most lab tests and many radiology procedures are "ordered" by the physician,
but performed elsewhere.

In this exercise, you will record the doctor's orders for several lab tests. There
are two ways to do this: by using the Entry Details Prefix field or by using the
Orders button on the Toolbar. In this step, you are going to use the Prefix field.

► Figure 5-10 **Recording the finding "An ECG was performed."**

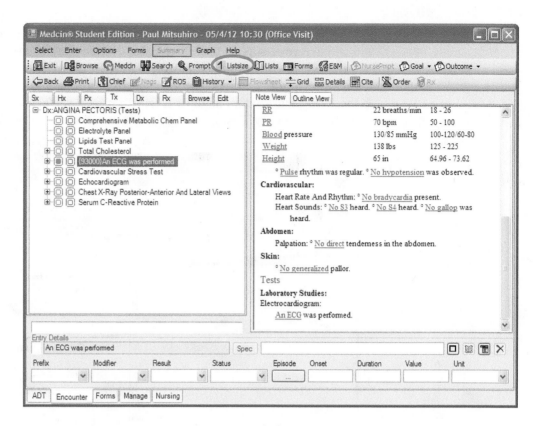

Locate and highlight the following test: "Electrolyte Panel."

With the finding Electrolyte Panel highlighted, click on the Prefix field at the bottom of the screen. A drop-down list will appear as shown in Figure 5-11. Locate and click on the word "ordered" in the list of prefixes.

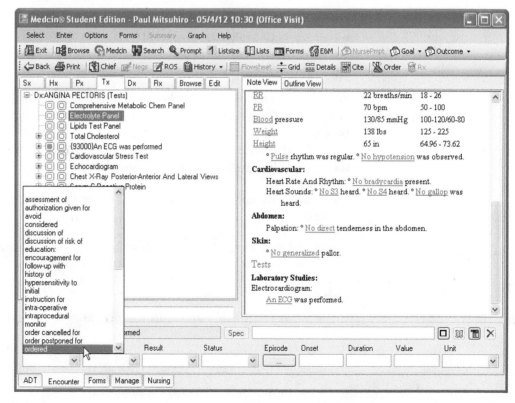

► Figure 5-11 **Drop-down list of the Prefix field used to order the "Electrolyte Panel."**

Step 15

Compare your screen to Figure 5-12. Notice that when you added the prefix "ordered" to the finding "Electrolyte Panel," it not only changed the meaning in the description, but also put the test in a different encounter note category than the ECG test. Medcin assigns a test that was performed or has a result status to the category of Tests, but assigns a test that is ordered to the category Plan.

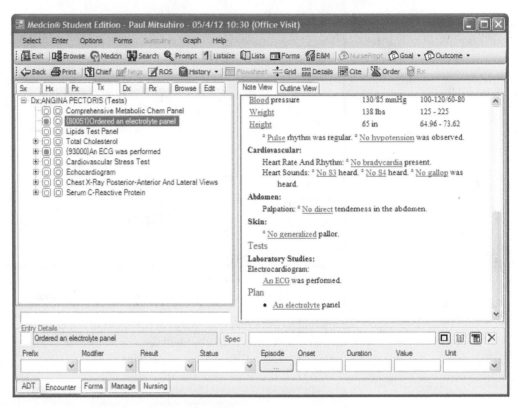

► Figure 5-12 **Electrolyte Panel ordered.**

Step 16

You can see that the method of ordering requires multiple clicks of the mouse. However, orders can be easily accomplished in a single step by using the Order button on the Toolbar. To order a test using the Order button, you need only highlight the finding and click the Order button. You do not have to click either the red or blue button for the finding.

Locate and click on the description "Lipids Test Panel" to highlight it (as shown in Figure 5-13).

Locate and click on the button labeled "Orders" in the Toolbar at the top of your screen. The Order icon resembles a lab beaker and test tube.

Step 17

Using what you have learned in the previous step, order an additional test and an x-ray:

Highlight the following findings and click on the Order button in the Toolbar for each:

        🔬 (order button) Total Cholesterol

        🔬 (order button) Chest X-Ray Posterior-Anterior and Lateral Views

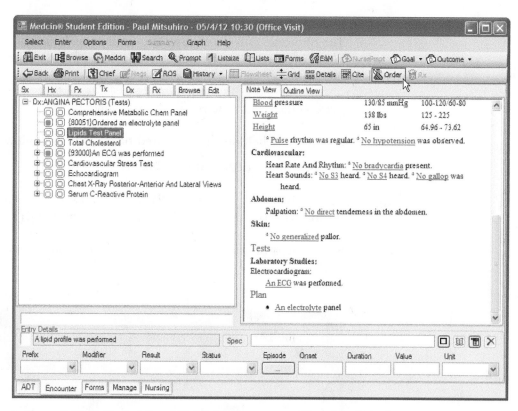

▶ Figure 5-13 **Lipids Test Panel highlighted; mouse positioned on Order button.**

Compare your screen to Figure 5-14. From this example, you can see the advantage of using Toolbar buttons for orders. Other Toolbar buttons are used for History items and prescriptions, as you will learn in subsequent exercises.

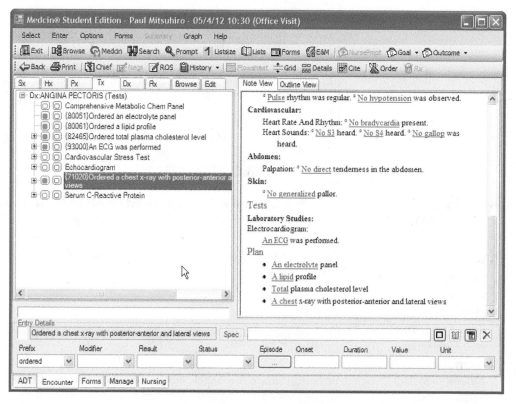

▶ Figure 5-14 **Tests and x-rays ordered using the Order button.**

Step 18

The clinician will determine the final assessment after the complete workup later this week. Therefore, the diagnosis at this time will be "possible angina pectoris."

Click on the Dx tab and record the assessment.

Locate and click on the indicated button for the following finding:

● (red button) Angina Pectoris

Locate the Prefix field in the Entry Details section. Click the mouse on the button with the down arrow within the Prefix field.

Scroll the drop-down list to locate and click on the word "possible," as shown in Figure 5-15.

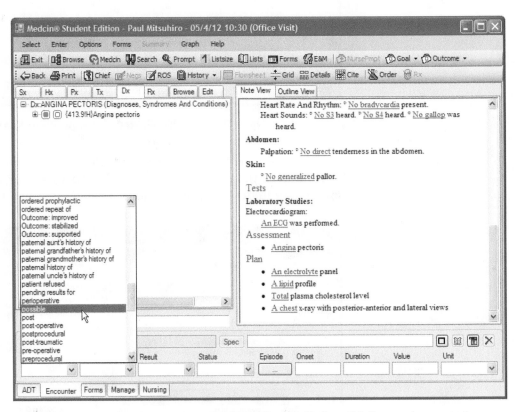

▶ Figure 5-15 **Dx tab with drop-down list for adding Prefix "possible" to angina pectoris.**

This completes Mr. Mitsuhiro's preliminary visit. Print your completed encounter note.

Step 19

Click on the Print button on the Toolbar at the top of your screen to invoke the Print Data window.

Be certain there is a check mark in the box next to "Current Encounter" and then click on the appropriate button to either print or export a file, as directed by your instructor.

Compare your printout or exported file to Figure 5-16. If it is correct, hand it in to your instructor. If there are any differences (other than the date and patient age), review the previous steps in the exercise and find your error.

Paul Mitsuhiro

Student: *your name or ID here*
Patient: Paul Mitsuhiro: M: 11/12/1962: 5/04/2012 10:30 AM
Chief complaint
The Chief Complaint is: Suspected Angina.
History of present illness
    Paul Mitsuhiro is a 49 year old male.
    He reported: Jaw pain during exercise.
    No chest pain or discomfort. No dyspnea.
Past medical/surgical history
Diagnosis History:
    No hypertension.
    No diabetes mellitus
Personal history
    Behavioral: Not a current smoker.
Physical findings
Vital Signs:

Vital Signs/Measurements	Value	Normal Range
Oral temperature	98.6 F	97.6 - 99.6
RR	22 breaths/min	18 - 26
PR	70 bpm	50 - 100
Blood pressure	130/85 mmHg	100-120/60-80
Weight	138 lbs	125 - 225
Height	65 in	64.96 - 73.62

° Pulse rhythm was regular. ° No hypotension was observed.
Cardiovascular:
    Heart Rate and Rhythm: ° No bradycardia present.
    Heart Sounds: ° No S3 heard. ° No S4 heard. ° No gallop was heard.
Abdomen:
    Palpation: ° No direct tenderness in the abdomen.
Skin:
    ° No generalized pallor.
Tests
Laboratory Studies:
    Electrocardiogram:
    An ECG was performed.
Assessment
- Possible angina pectoris
Plan
- An electrolyte panel
- A lipid profile
- Total plasma cholesterol level
- A chest x-ray with posterior-anterior and lateral views

▶ **Figure 5-16 Printed encounter note with angina orders for Paul Mitsuhiro.**

Recording Orders in the Student Edition

Thus far in this chapter, you have learned to record lab and x-ray orders. In subsequent chapters you will learn how to record medication orders and order other tests. Though you may not be a healthcare provider who writes medical orders, there are a number of reasons we include orders in this course:

1. **Orders are an essential component of any patient chart and a key point identified by the IOM, Leapfrog, and the HITECH act as discussed in Chapter 1.**
2. **Exercises that include orders and results offer you a more realistic experience of the complete EHR.**
3. **Nurses, medical assistants, ward clerks, and other allied health professionals often enter verbal orders into an EHR on behalf of the ordering clinician.**

These exercises simulate the process of ordering and tracking lab results on a computer. However, the Student Edition does not contain a working electronic lab order system. You cannot use the Student Edition software to write or send actual orders to a lab; this ability would be inappropriate in a student edition.

Similarly, exercises in the next chapter include a simulation of writing prescriptions electronically. Again, the Student Edition does not contain a real electronic prescription system. You cannot use it to write or send actual prescriptions to a pharmacy; this also would be inappropriate in a student edition.

Critical Thinking Exercise 32: Ordering an X-Ray

Patient Manuel Lopez has injured his knee. Using what you have learned in this chapter, document his visit and the doctor's orders.

Step 1

If you have not already done so, start the Student Edition software.

Click Select on the Menu bar, and then click Patient.

In the Patient Selection window, locate and click on "Manuel Lopez."

Step 2

Click Select on the Menu bar, and then click New Encounter.

You may use the current the date and time for this exercise.

Select the reason "Office Visit" from the Reason drop-down list. Click on the OK button.

Step 3

Enter the chief complaint by locating the button in the Toolbar labeled "Chief" and clicking on it.

In the dialog window that opens, type **Twisted his knee**.

Click on the button labeled "Close the note form."

Step 4

Locate and click on the Search button on the Toolbar near the top of the screen. (The search button was highlighted orange in Figure 5-5.)

Click your mouse in the Search String field and enter the medical term **knee sprain**. Verify that you have spelled this correctly, and then click the button in the box labeled "Search."

If you see the message "nothing found to match search," repeat step 4 and verify that you have spelled the medical term correctly.

Step 5

Locate and click on the Prompt button on the Toolbar near the top of the screen. (The Prompt button was circled in red in Figure 5-7.)

Step 6

If the nomenclature pane is not automatically on the Symptoms (Sx) tab, click the Sx tab.

Locate "Joint pain localized in the knee" and click on the small plus sign.

Locate and click on the following findings:

● (red button) Right

Scroll the nomenclature pane to locate and click on the following finding:

● (red button) Joint swelling of the lateral right knee

Step 7

Click the Hx tab.

Click on the small plus sign next to "Reported trauma to the knee."

Locate and click on the following finding:

● (red button) Due to twisting

Step 8

Click the Px tab.

Locate "Knee swelling" and click on the small plus sign.

Locate and click on the following finding:

● (red button) Right

Scroll the list downward to locate "Knee tenderness on palpitation" and click on the small plus sign.

Locate and click on the following finding:

● (red button) Right Knee

Step 9

Click the Dx tab.

Locate and click on the following finding:

● (red button) Knee sprain

Step 10

Click the Tx tab.

Locate, highlight, and order the following finding:

         (order button) X-Ray Knee w/oblique 3 or more views

Step 11

Click the Rx tab.

If the list size is not 1, click the Listsize button on the Toolbar until the list size is "1."

Locate and click on the following findings:

         ● (red button) Ordered reduced physical activity
         ● (red button) Ordered Ace bandage

! **Alert**

Do not close or exit the encounter until you have a printed copy in your hand. *You will lose your work if you exit before printing.*

Step 12

Print your completed encounter note:

Click on the Print button on the Toolbar at the top of your screen to invoke the Print Data window.

Be certain there is a check mark in the box next to "Current Encounter" and then click on the appropriate button to either print or export a file, as directed by your instructor.

Compare your printout or file output to Figure 5-17. If it is correct, hand it in to your instructor. If there are any differences, review the previous steps in the exercise and find your error.

Manuel Lopez   Page 1 of 1

Student: *your name or ID here*
Patient: Manuel Lopez: M: 7/30/1984: 5/08/2012 09:30 AM
Chief complaint
The Chief Complaint is: Twisted his knee.
History of present illness
     Manuel Lopez is a 27 year old male.
     He reported: Right knee joint pain and knee joint swelling on the right laterally.
Past medical/surgical history
Reported History:
     Physical Trauma: Trauma to the knee due to twisting.
Physical findings
Musculoskeletal System:
     Knee:
     Right Knee: • Swelling. • Tenderness on palpation.
Assessment
     • Knee sprain
Plan
       • X-rays of the knee with oblique(s), three or more views
       • Reduced physical activity
       • Ace bandage

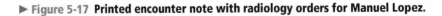

▶ Figure 5-17 **Printed encounter note with radiology orders for Manuel Lopez.**

Chapter Five Summary

In this chapter you learned to use the Search and Prompt features and two ways of recording a clinician's orders. You also learned more about the Medcin Toolbar.

Toolbar The Toolbar is used to quickly access commonly used functions. The Toolbar has two rows of icon buttons that help you in three different ways:

1. Some buttons eliminate the need to access the menu for frequently used items.

2. Other buttons control the behavior or look of the panes in the Medcin window.

3. Several buttons set the prefix on a finding so you don't have to go to the Entry Details fields to do it.

Search The Search function provides a quick way to locate a desired finding in the nomenclature. Medcin addresses semantic differences in medical terms in three ways:

1. Search performs automatic word completion, so if you search for *knee* but the finding is for *knees*, the system will still find it.

2. Medcin includes an extensive list of synonyms that are used in an alternate word search. For example, if you search for *knee injury*, the search results will also include findings for *knee burns*, *knee trauma*, and *fractured patella*, among others.

3. Search identifies related findings in other tabs so that when you search for a word or phrase in a particular tab, related findings are automatically available in the other tabs. This means that when you are using search while documenting a patient exam, as you continue through the exam, the other tabs will already have findings that you may need.

Search is not designed to find every instance that contains the words being searched because the search results would often have too many findings. Instead, search finds and displays the highest level match but does not list all the expanded findings below it.

Prompt The term *Prompt* is short for "prompt with current finding." Prompt generates a list of findings that are clinically related to the finding currently highlighted.

The prompt list that is displayed is shorter than the full nomenclature, containing only relevant findings, which makes it easier to read and navigate. The list generated by the prompt feature populates all of the applicable tabs, creating shorter lists of any relevant findings in each tab (Sx, Hx, Px, Tx, Dx, and Rx).

Listsize The List Size function changes the quantity of findings displayed in a list.

As you continue through the course, you can refer to the Toolbar reference at the beginning of this chapter when you need to remember the function of a particular button. Refer to the guided exercises listed below if you need to remember how to perform a particular task.

Task	Exercise	Page
Guide to Toolbar buttons	n/a	117
Search for a finding in the nomenclature	30	119
Prompt (locate findings related to highlighted finding)	30	119
Record orders (or change order status) using the drop-down list	31	126
Record orders using the Orders button on the Toolbar	31	126

Testing Your Knowledge of Chapter 5

You may run the Medcin Student Edition software and use your mouse on the screen to answer the following questions:

1. Describe how to record a test that was ordered and describe how to record a test that was performed.

2. How do you indicate a "possible" diagnosis?

Describe the function of each of the following buttons on the Toolbar:

3. Exit

4. Browse

5. Chief

6. Search

7. Order

8. Print

9. Prompt

10. When you click the Prompt button, what list will be generated?

11. How do you change the numbers on the Listsize button and what do the numbers do?

Circle True or False for the following statements:

12. Orders are an essential component of any patient chart.

    True   False

13. Medical assistants sometimes enter verbal orders into an EHR on behalf of the ordering clinician.

    True   False

14. The use of CPOE, in conjunction with an EHR, improves clinician productivity.

    True   False

15. In this chapter, you should have produced two narrative documents of patient encounters, which you printed. If you have not already done so, hand these in to your instructor with this test. The printed encounter notes will count as a portion of your grade.

Learning to Use Lists

Learning Outcomes

After completing this chapter, you should be able to:

◆ Understand how lists of findings can speed data entry

◆ Know how to use the Lists Manager to load lists

◆ Record orders for tests and therapies

◆ Record prescriptions

Shortcuts That Increase Speed for Routine Encounters

The Search feature is fine for quickly locating findings related to anything that you do not see on a regular basis. However, most medical offices see a lot of patients with the same conditions. In these cases physicians tend to perform the same type of exam, look for the same findings, order the same tests, and prescribe from a short list of treatments recommended for the condition. Therefore, it is logical for the practice to create shorter, quicker methods of entering the data by the type of exam or condition.

For example, imagine a pediatrician who treats many children with earaches (otitis media) and that each time the patient's chief complaint was earache the system could magically present the findings typically used to document the visit.

In this chapter and the next, we will explore two features that are used extensively in EHR systems, lists and forms. These features are templates that display findings that the clinician uses most frequently for different types of conditions or diseases so that the encounter can be documented with minimal navigation or searching.

The Concept of Lists

You may not have heard the term *lists* used in the context of an EHR, but the concept should be very familiar to you because you have been scrolling and navigating the list of findings since Chapter 3. In the previous chapter, the Prompt function created a short list of findings that were relevant to the words for which you were searching. The advantage of using these short lists is that they behave just like lists in the full Medcin nomenclature except that they display only the desired subset of findings. The list can (and usually does) contain findings in every tab. This means that time savings are realized throughout documentation of the encounter.

While using a list, if a finding is needed that is not on the list, the provider can instantly switch to the full hierarchy of Medcin findings and then back to the list.

Although lists are sometimes limited to one particular condition such as otitis media, this is not a rule; it is a convenience factor because shorter lists mean less scrolling. Lists are flexible and can contain as many findings as necessary to document a typical visit.

With some types of symptoms, the assessment could be one of several possible diagnoses. For example, adult upper respiratory infections could be the result of rhinitis, sinusitis, or bronchitis. Therefore, a list with more findings reduces the possibility that the provider will need to switch to browsing the full nomenclature.

A good example of a multiple diagnosis type of list is the one used for the following exercise. During the cold and flu season, medical clinics and primary care physicians often see many patients with upper respiratory infections (URIs). Therefore, a list of findings for adults presenting with URI symptoms can really speed the documentation process.

Guided Exercise 33: Using an Adult URI List

In this exercise, you will learn to use the List feature as well as several additional buttons on the Toolbar.

Carrie Cook comes to the office complaining of sinus pain, stuffiness, and a runny nose. She says she has caught her husband's "bug." The medical practice has created a list of findings typically used for this type of visit. They have named it "Adult URI."

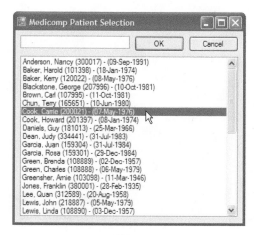

► Figure 6-1 **Selecting Carrie Cook from the Patient Selection window.**

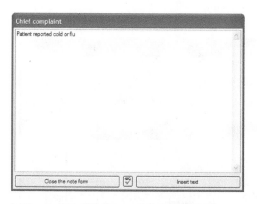

► Figure 6-2 **Chief complaint window for "Patient reported cold or flu."**

Step 1

If you have not already done so, start the Student Edition software.

Click Select on the Menu bar, and then click Patient.

In the Patient Selection window, locate and click on "Carrie Cook" as shown in Figure 6-1.

Step 2

Click Select on the Menu bar, and then click New Encounter.

Use the current date and time. Select the reason "10 Minute Visit." Click on the OK button.

Step 3

Enter the chief complaint by locating the button in the Toolbar labeled "Chief" and clicking on it.

In the dialog window that opens, type **Patient reported cold or flu.**

Compare your screen to Figure 6-2 before clicking on the button labeled "Close the note form."

Step 4

In this exercise, the medical assistant will begin the visit by taking Carrie Cook's vital signs.

Use the form labeled "Vitals," which you will select from the Forms Manager, as you have done in previous exercises.

Enter Ms. Cook's vital signs in the corresponding fields on the form as follows:

Temperature:	**99**
Respiration:	**16**
Pulse:	**78**
BP:	**120/80**
Height:	**60**
Weight:	**100**

When you have finished, compare your screen to Figure 6-3 and, when it is correct, click on the Encounter tab at the bottom of the screen.

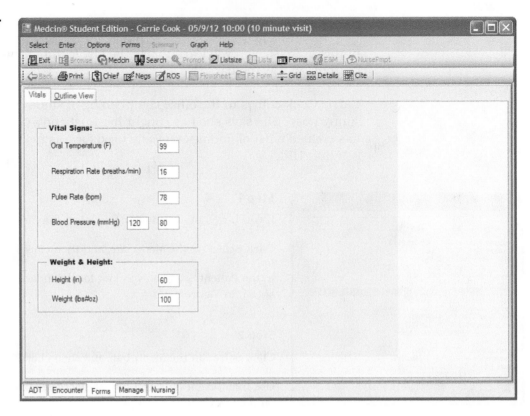

Step 5

Because the patient reported cold or flu symptoms, we will use a list created for this type of encounter:

Locate and click on the Lists button in the Toolbar at the top of your screen (highlighted orange in Figure 6-4). The icon resembles an open book.

► Figure 6-4 **Select Adult URI from Lists Manager window (invoked by Lists button.)**

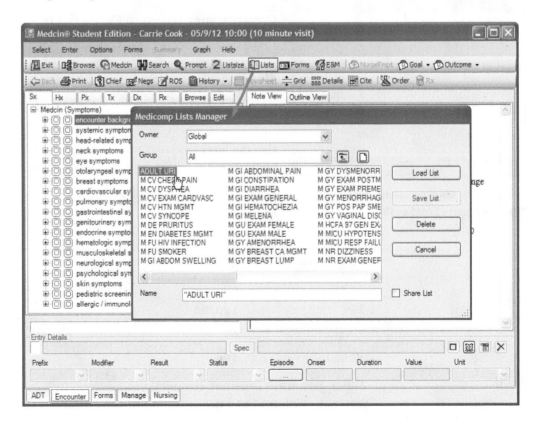

The Lists Manager window will be invoked. The Lists Manager displays the various lists available to providers in the practice. Two fields at the top of the screen organize the display of list names, filtering them by Owner and Group.

As we discussed earlier in this section, clinicians also can create personal copies of lists customized to their style of practice. The Owner field allows clinicians to quickly find their customized lists by changing the field from "Global" to "Personal."

Lists also can be assigned to Groups, which helps organize them by body system, disease, type of encounter, or any other criteria the practice desires. The Group field allows a user to quickly find a list by limiting the display to a desired group. Note that the Student Edition has two groups, "All" and "Student Edition."

Locate and highlight the list named Adult URI, which is the first list in the window. Click your mouse on the button labeled "Load List."

▶ Figure 6-5 **Symptoms on the Adult URI List. HPI section is circled in red.**

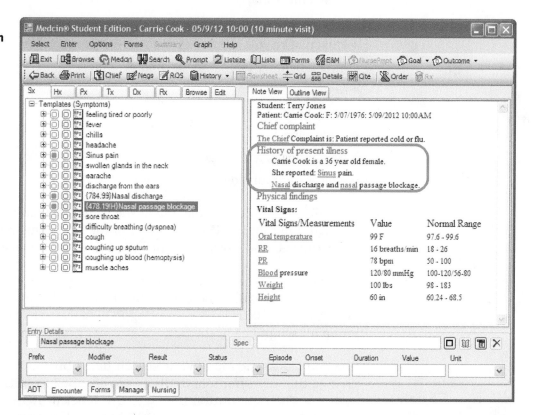

Step 6

Notice that the normal display of the Medcin nomenclature in the left pane has been replaced with a list of symptoms that patients with upper respiratory infections are likely to report. Notice that the title of the first line "Templates (Symptoms)" indicates that the findings are limited by a list (referred to in the left pane as a "Template"). You will also notice a special HPI button next to each finding, this will be explained in a moment.

Locate and click on the following symptom findings:

- (red button) Sinus pain
- (red button) Nasal discharge
- (red button) Nasal blockage (from stuffiness)

Compare your screen to Figure 6-5. Before proceeding, notice that symptoms reported by the patient have been documented in the "History of present illness" or "HPI" section in the encounter note (circled in red).

Step 7

The term *review of systems* (ROS) refers to a way of organizing an exam by body systems starting from the head down. You may be familiar with the body systems from anatomy and physiology or other medical classes. The body systems in a standard ROS are:

- Constitutional symptoms
- HEENT (head, eyes, ears, nose, mouth, throat)
- Cardiovascular
- Respiratory
- Gastrointestinal
- Genitourinary
- Musculoskeletal
- Integumentary (skin and/or breast)
- Neurologic
- Psychiatric
- Endocrine
- Hematologic/lymphatic
- Allergic/immunologic.

Typically, a provider will document the symptoms directly related to the chief complaint in the HPI. The remainder of the symptoms review is to rule out other causes. It is typically documented in a "Review of systems" or "ROS."

In Chapter 8, you will learn about the CMS coding guidelines used to determine the correct Evaluation and Management code for billing. Because the CMS guidelines have specific rules for counting ROS body systems, it is not advisable to group all symptoms in the HPI.

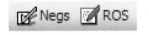

▶ Figure 6-6 **Auto Negative (Negs) and Review of Systems (ROS) buttons.**

The Toolbar at the top of your screen has a button that can be used to change the way symptom findings are grouped from HPI into a review of systems. The right button in Figure 6-6 labeled "ROS" toggles between on and off. When you click on the ROS button, it changes from blue to orange. This indicates that the ROS grouping is on. If you click on the button again, it will change back to its original color, blue. This indicates that the ROS grouping is off.

Locate and click on the ROS button. It will turn orange as shown in Figure 6-7. When you click on symptom findings while the ROS button is orange, the findings selected will be placed in the Review of systems group.

Step 8

Verify the ROS button is orange, then locate and click on the following finding:

- (blue button) Headache

► **Figure 6-7 Symptom: "No headache" in "Review of systems" group (circled in red).**

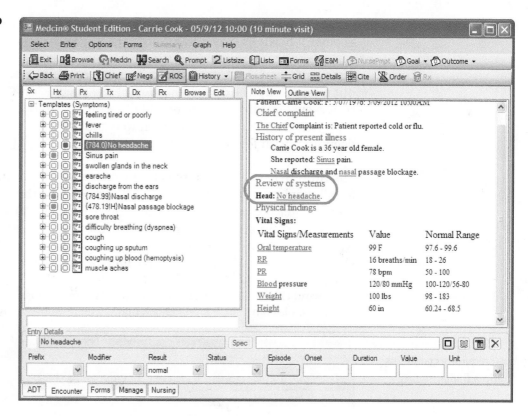

Compare your screen to Figure 6-7. Notice that the finding "No headache" was placed in a new group "Review of systems" that was created in the note (shown circled in red).

The small HPI button next to each finding in the nomenclature pane would allow a user to switch an individual finding from HPI to ROS without using the ROS button on the Toolbar. You will not be using the button on the individual findings in this exercise.

The differences between the actions of these two buttons are as follows:

◆ The ROS button on the Toolbar applies to all symptoms selected while the button is on (orange.)
◆ The HPI/ROS button on an individual finding affects only the selected finding and only affects it when the Toolbar ROS button is off (blue).
◆ The HPI/ROS button on individual findings is only available on the Sx tab, and only when a list is loaded.
◆ The ROS button on the Toolbar is available anytime you are on the Sx tab.

Step 9

Frequently, most of the symptoms in the ROS will be negative, because they were not reported by the patient in the HPI. Using a list such as Adult URI, you could quickly go down the list clicking a blue button on each of the remaining findings. However, that would still be a lot of mouse clicks.

Fortunately, the Toolbar has another button, labeled "Negs" for "Auto Negative" that is used to speed up the documentation process. When the clinician has clicked a red or blue button for all of the relevant positive findings, the remainder of the list can be set to the negative with one click on the "Negs" button on the Toolbar (shown enlarged in Figure 6-6).

The purpose of the Auto Negative feature is not to shortcut the exam process, but to speed up the documentation of the encounter. Clinicians find they can review systems much more quickly than they can document each finding. The Auto Negative feature allows them to complete this portion of the encounter document with fewer clicks.

The Auto Negative feature selects the "normal" button (usually the blue button) for all displayed findings that are not already set. The user can modify any finding after the process is finished. Because all of the findings displayed in the current tab are automatically selected, the Auto Negative feature works best with lists or forms because the list is already limited to findings the clinician would normally use in a particular type of encounter.

Locate and click on the button labeled "Negs" in the Toolbar at the top of your screen. The icon resembles a box with a teal check mark. The Negs button is highlighted in Figure 6-8.

▶ Figure 6-8 **Auto Negative button quickly completes multiple findings.**

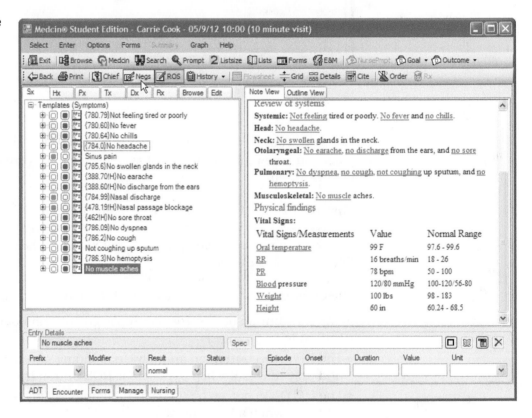

All symptoms that have not previously been selected have automatically had their blue buttons selected. Notice how quickly the documentation process was completed.

Compare the encounter notes on your screen with Figure 6-8. (You may need to scroll the right pane upward to see the full effect.) Notice that the three findings with red buttons were not altered.

The Auto Negative function will record the findings according to the state of the ROS button. Because the ROS button was orange, the additional symptoms were recorded in the Review of Symptoms group, not the HPI group.

Step 10

Although all unselected symptoms findings were set with the Auto Negative feature, they can be changed by the user at any time while documenting the encounter. Note that Ms. Cook's temperature is 99°F. Therefore, she has a slight fever. You can update the encounter note in this way:

Locate and click on the following finding:

● (red button) No Fever

The finding will change to "Fever."

With the finding still highlighted, click your mouse on the button with the down arrow in the Entry Details Modifier field to display a drop-down list (as shown in Figure 6-9).

Scroll the list of modifiers until you locate the word "Mild" and click on it.

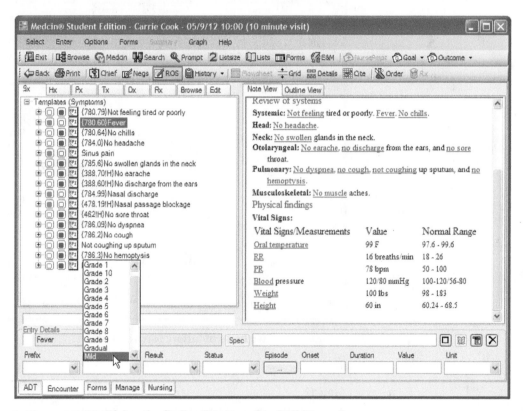

▶ Figure 6-9 **Modifying the finding "No Fever" to "Mild Fever."**

Step 11

Next, click on the Hx tab to enter the patient's history. Note that the "Negs" button is grayed out. The Auto Negative button is only available on the Sx (Symptoms) and Px (Physical Exam) tabs.

You will recall from previous exercises that the Hx tab normally has a lot of findings, but because you are using a list, only those findings related to Adult URI are displayed. This makes navigation of the list quicker because it is shorter.

Locate and click on the following history findings:

- (red button) Recent upper respiratory infection (URI)
- (blue button) Allergies
- (blue button) Taking medication
- (blue button) current smoker

Note that Allergy findings are in their own group below Physical Exam. Now scroll your screen upward. Compare your screen to the Reported History circled in red in Figure 6-10. Note that even though the findings were listed together in the left pane, they were actually from three different history groups Past Medical History, Social History (Behavioral), and Allergies.

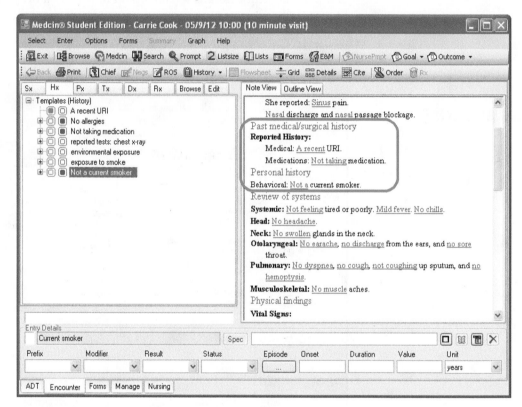

▶ Figure 6-10 **Two types of history (circled in red).**

Step 12

Click on the Px tab to document the physical exam. Note that the Negs button in the Toolbar is available when you are on this tab.

Locate and click on the following Physical Exam findings:

- (blue button) Both tympanic membranes were examined
- (red button) Nasal discharge purulent
- (red button) Sinus tenderness

Now locate the button labeled "Negs" in the Toolbar and click it once.

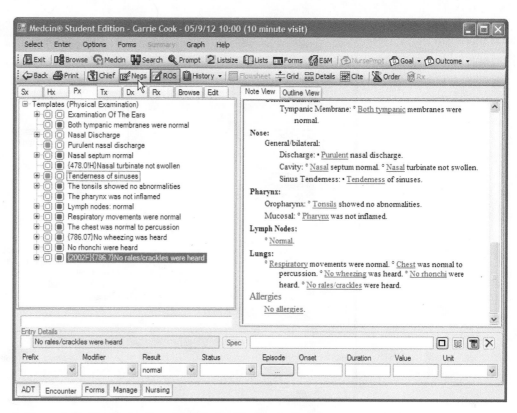

▶ Figure 6-11 **Physical exam completed using Neg button.**

Compare your screen to Figure 6-11. Notice that the first and third findings (ears and nasal discharge) were not set. This because the Auto Negative feature correctly determined that the tympanic membrane finding was an examination of the ears, and the purulent discharge finding was a refinement of the nasal discharge finding. Note also that although the ROS button may still be orange on your Toolbar, ROS has no effect in the Px tab.

Step 13

The clinician has determined that the patient has acute sinusitis. Click on the Dx tab and notice that the Adult URI list contains only diagnoses that the practice has decided are likely to present for this type of condition.

Locate and click on the following finding:

● (red button) Sinusitis Acute

Compare your screen to Figure 6-12.

► Figure 6-12 **Assessment:**
Acute sinusitis.

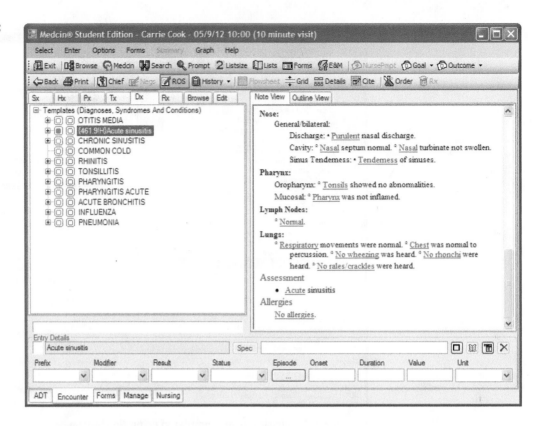

► Figure 6-13 **Fluids ordered**
for Carrie Cook.

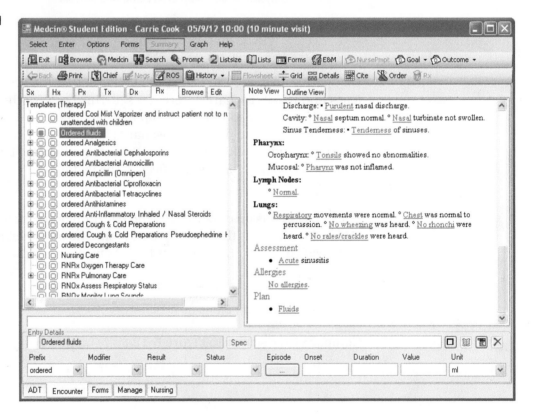

Step 14

Click on the Rx tab and again appreciate the fact that the tab contains only types of treatments that the practice is likely to prescribe for an adult upper respiratory infection. The clinician is going to order fluids and an antibiotic.

Locate and click on the following finding:

- (red button) Fluids

Compare your screen to Figure 6-13.

Do not exit the program until you have completed the following exercise.

Guided Exercise 34: Recording Prescriptions in an EHR

Step 15

Locate the Prescription button in the Toolbar at the top of your screen. The button is labeled "Rx" and its icon resembles a small prescription bottle, but because the finding "Ordered Fluids" is still highlighted, the button will appear grayed out. The button is shown highlighted orange in Figure 6-14.

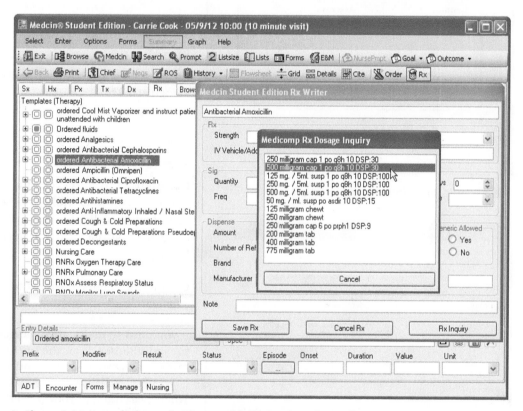

▶ Figure 6-14 **Prescription writer button (highlighted on the Toolbar) with Rx Dosage Inquiry window.**

Locate and highlight the finding "Antibacterial Amoxicillin." The button labeled "Rx" on the Toolbar will become available when you highlight the finding. The Prescription (Rx) button is enabled only when you are on the Rx tab and only if the highlighted finding is a medication.

With the finding "Antibacterial Amoxicillin" highlighted, click on the Prescription (Rx) button in the Toolbar. A simple Prescription Writer window will be invoked, as shown in Figure 6-14.

Step 16

When you clicked on the prescription (Rx) button and invoked the Prescription Writer window, the drug was automatically selected from the finding. A list of available dosages is automatically displayed. This is the "Sig"[1] information that the pharmacist will include on the label. It consists of the quantity prescribed, the number of times per day, capsules to take each time, number of days to take the drug, the total quantity prescribed, the number of refills allowed, and any free-text instructions to the patient. The list of available Sig choices makes writing the prescription very fast. It is found in virtually all commercial EHR prescription systems.

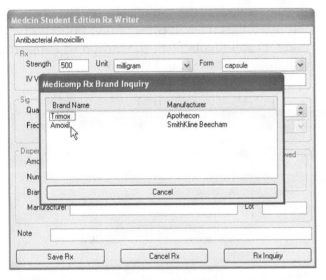

► Figure 6-15 **Prescription brand selection.**

Locate and click your mouse on the Sig: "500 milligram cap 1 po q8h 10 DSP:30," shown highlighted in Figure 6-14.

The next window displaying available brands (as shown in Figure 6-15) will be displayed automatically.

Step 17

Locate and click on "Amoxil SmithKline Beecham," as shown in Figure 6-15.

Step 18

Compare your screen to Figure 6-16. Locate the "Generic Allowed" field. The "Yes" and "No" buttons are used to indicate whether the pharmacist is allowed to substitute a generic drug for a prescribed brand.

Click in the small circle next to "Yes." This action fills in the small circle.

If you need to make any changes or corrections in the prescription, click on the button labeled "Rx Inquiry" to invoke the Dosage and Brand windows again.

When everything in your prescription screen matches Figure 6-16, click on the Save Rx button.

The prescription information will be written into the Plan section of the encounter note as shown in Figure 6-17.

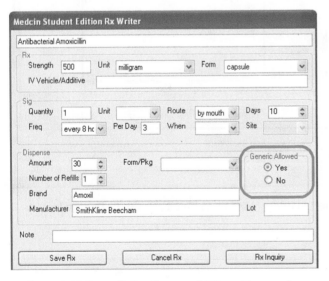

► Figure 6-16 **Prescription for amoxicillin, with generic choices circled in red.**

In this exercise you learned to use the List feature as well as the ROS and Auto Negative buttons. You also learned to use the Modifier field and record a prescription.

---

[1]Sig, from the Latin *signa*, are instructions for labeling a prescription.

► Figure 6-17 Completed Adult URI encounter for Carrie Cook.

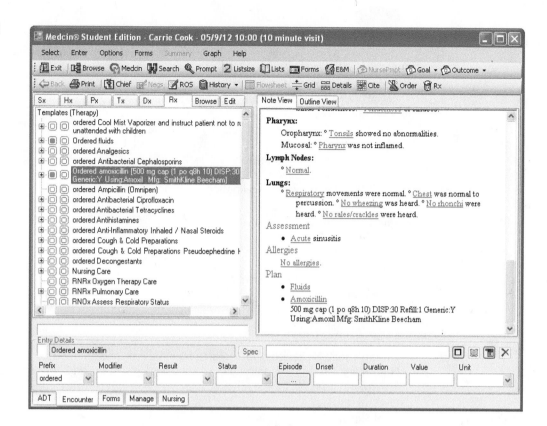

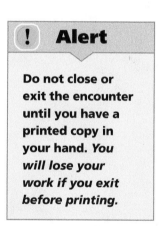

Alert

Do not close or exit the encounter until you have a printed copy in your hand. *You will lose your work if you exit before printing.*

Step 19

Click on the Print button on the Toolbar at the top of your screen to invoke the Print Data window.

Be certain there is a check mark in the box next to "Current Encounter" and then click on the appropriate button to either print or export a file, as directed by your instructor.

Compare your printout or file output to Figure 6-18. If it is correct, hand it in to your instructor. If there are any differences (other than the date and patient age), review the previous steps in the exercise and find your error.

Critical Thinking Exercise 35: Timed Experiment

Now that you have learned that the Lists and Auto Negative features can help you enter EHR data more quickly, prove it to yourself with this exercise. In Chapter 4, you documented a visit for an adult URI for Ms. Cook's husband, Howard Cook. In this exercise he is returning because his condition has not improved. You are going to document a visit very similar to his previous visit, but this time using what you have learned about lists.

Step 1

Look at the clock and write down the current time.

If you have not already done so, start the Student Edition software.

Click Select on the Menu bar, and then click Patient.

In the Patient Selection window, locate and click on "Howard Cook."

Student: *your name or ID here*
Patient: Carrie Cook: F: 5/07/1976: 5/09/2012 10:00 AM

Chief complaint

The Chief Complaint is: Patient reported cold or flu.

History of present illness

Carrie Cook is a 36 year old female.
She reported: Sinus pain.
Nasal discharge and nasal passage blockage.

Past medical/surgical history

Reported History:
Medical: A recent URI.
Medications: Not taking medication.

Personal history

Behavioral: Not a current smoker.

Review of systems

Systemic: Not feeling tired or poorly. Mild fever. No chills.
Head: No headache.
Neck: No swollen glands in the neck.
Otolaryngeal: No earache, no discharge from the ears, and no sore throat.
Pulmonary: No dyspnea, no cough, not coughing up sputum, and no hemoptysis.
Musculoskeletal: No muscle aches.

Physical findings

Vital Signs:

Vital Signs/Measurements	Value	Normal Range
Oral temperature	99 F	97.6 - 99.6
RR	16 breaths/min	18 - 26
PR	78 bpm	50 - 100
Blood pressure	120/80 mmHg	100-120/56-80
Weight	100 lbs	98 - 183
Height	60 in	60.24 - 68.5

Ears:
General/bilateral:
Tympanic Membrane: ° Both tympanic membranes were normal.
Nose:
General/bilateral:
Discharge: • Purulent nasal discharge.
Cavity: ° Nasal septum normal. ° Nasal turbinate not swollen.
Sinus Tenderness: • Tenderness of sinuses.
Pharynx:
Oropharynx: ° Tonsils showed no abnormalities.
Mucosal: ° Pharynx was not inflamed.
Lymph Nodes:
° Normal.
Lungs:
° Respiratory movements were normal. ° Chest was normal to percussion. ° No wheezing was heard. ° No rhonchi were heard. ° No rales/crackles were heard.

Assessment

• Acute sinusitis

Allergies

No allergies.

Plan

• Fluids
• Amoxicillin
500 mg cap (1 po q8h 10) DISP:30 Refill:1 Generic:Y Using:Amoxil Mfg: SmithKline Beecham

▶ **Figure 6-18 Printed encounter note (with prescription) for Carrie Cook.**

Step 2

Click Select on the Menu bar, and then click New Encounter.

Select the reason "10 minute visit" from the Reason drop-down list.

Make sure you have selected the reason correctly. You may use the current date for this exercise.

Step 3

Enter the chief complaint by locating the button in the Toolbar labeled "Chief" and clicking on it.

In the dialog window that opens, type **Return visit for cold**.

Click on the button labeled "Close the note form."

Step 4

Click on the Forms tab at the bottom of the window.

Click on the Forms button on the Toolbar to invoke the Forms Manager window.

Select the form labeled "Vitals." Enter Howard Cook's vital signs in the corresponding fields on the form as follows:

Temperature:	**99.7**
Respiration:	**20**
Pulse:	**60**
BP:	**120/80**
Height:	**72**
Weight:	**175**

When you have finished, click on the Encounter tab at the bottom of the screen.

Step 5

Locate and click on the Lists button in the Toolbar at the top of your screen (highlighted orange in Figure 6-4). The Lists Manager window will be invoked.

Locate and highlight the list named Adult URI. Click your mouse on the button labeled "Load List."

Step 6

Verify that the first line of the Medcin Nomenclature in the left pane reads: "Templates (Symptoms)."

Locate and click on the following symptom findings:

- (red button) Headache
- (red button) Sinus pain
- (red button) Nasal discharge
- (red button) Nasal passage blockage (stuffiness)

Step 7

Expand the list of findings by clicking the small plus sign next to "Nasal discharge."

Locate and click on the following symptom findings:

- (red button) recurs frequently

Step 8

Howard's vital signs show a mild fever.

Locate a click on the following symptom finding:

- (red button) Fever

Modify the finding "Fever" by clicking the down arrow in the Entry Details Modifier field to display a drop-down list. Scroll the list of modifiers until you locate the word "Mild" and click on it.

The description should change to "Mild Fever."

Step 9

Locate and click on the ROS button on the Toolbar. The ROS button should change color from blue to orange.

Verify the ROS button is orange, then locate and click on the button labeled "Negs" in the Toolbar at the top of your screen. (The Negs button is highlighted in Figure 6-8.)

Step 10

Click on the Hx tab to enter the patient's history.

Locate and click on the following history findings:

- (red button) Recent upper respiratory infection (URI)
- (blue button) Allergies
- (blue button) current smoker

Locate "taking medications" and expand the tree by clicking the small plus sign.

Scroll the screen to locate and expand the tree for "over-the-counter."

Locate and click the following finding:

- (red button) for colds

Step 11

Click on the Px tab to document the physical exam.

Locate and click on the following Physical Exam findings.

- (blue button) Both tympanic membranes were examined
- (red button) Nasal discharge
- (red button) Nasal discharge purulent
- (red button) Sinus tenderness

Step 12

Now locate the button labeled "Negs" in the Toolbar and click it once.

Step 13

The clinician has determined that Howard Cook has acute sinusitis.

Click on the Dx tab and then locate and click on the following finding:

- (red button) Sinusitis Acute

Step 14

The clinician is going to order fluids and an antibiotic.

Click on the Rx tab and then locate and click on the following finding:

  ● (red button) Fluids

Step 15

Locate and highlight the finding "Antibacterial Amoxicillin."

Locate and click on the button labeled Rx on the Toolbar. (The Rx button is highlighted in Figure 6-14.)

The Prescription Writer window will be invoked.

Step 16

Locate and click your mouse on the Sig: "500 milligram cap 1 po q8h 10 DSP:30."

The next window displaying available brands (as shown in Figure 6-15) will be displayed automatically.

Step 17

Locate and click on "Amoxil SmithKline Beecham."

Step 18

Locate the "Generic Allowed" fields. Click in the small circle next to "Yes." This action fills in the small circle.

Click on the button labeled "Save Rx."

> **! Alert**
>
> Do not close or exit the encounter until you have a printed copy in your hand. *You will lose your work if you exit before printing.*

Step 19

Look at the clock and write down the time you completed the encounter note. Were you surprised how quickly you completed the entire encounter note?

Click on the Print button on the Toolbar at the top of your screen to invoke the Print Data window.

Be certain there is a check mark in the box next to "Current Encounter" and then click on the appropriate button to either print or export a file, as directed by your instructor.

If you are printing your work, write your start and stop time on your printed encounter note.

Compare your printout or file output to Figure 6-19. If it is correct, hand it in to your instructor. If there are any differences (other than the date and patient age), review the previous steps in the exercise and find your error.

Student: *your name or ID here*
Patient: Howard Cook: M: 1/08/1974: 5/09/2012 10:15 AM
Chief complaint
The Chief Complaint is: Return visit for cold.
History of present illness
      Howard Cook is a 38 year old male.
      He reported: Mild fever.
      Headache and sinus pain.
      Nasal discharge recurs frequently and nasal passage blockage.
Past medical/surgical history
Reported History:
      Medical: A recent URI.
      Medications: Taking OTC cold medication.
Personal history
      Behavioral: Not a current smoker.
Review of systems
Systemic: Not feeling tired or poorly. No chills.
Neck: No swollen glands in the neck.
Otolaryngeal: No earache, no discharge from the ears, and no sore throat.
Pulmonary: No dyspnea, no cough, not coughing up sputum, and no hemoptysis.
Musculoskeletal: No muscle aches.
Physical findings
Vital Signs:

Vital Signs/Measurements	Value	Normal Range
Oral temperature	99.7 F	97.6 - 99.6
RR	20 breaths/min	18 - 26
PR	60 bpm	50 - 100
Blood pressure	120/80 mmHg	100-120/56-80
Weight	175 lbs	125 - 225
Height	72 in	65.35 - 74.02

Ears:
      General/bilateral:
        ° Ears: normal.
Nose:
      General/bilateral:
        Discharge: • Nasal discharge seen. • Purulent nasal discharge.
        Cavity: ° Nasal septum normal. ° Nasal turbinate not swollen.
        Sinus Tenderness: • Tenderness of sinuses.
Pharynx:
      Oropharynx: ° Tonsils showed no abnormalities.
      Mucosal: ° Pharynx was not inflamed.
Lymph Nodes:
      ° Normal.
Lungs:
      ° Respiratory movements were normal. ° Chest was normal to percussion. ° No wheezing was heard. ° No rhonchi were heard. ° No rales/crackles were heard.
Assessment
      • Acute sinusitis
Allergies
      No allergies.
Plan
      • Fluids
      • Amoxicillin
      500 mg cap (1 po q8h 10) DISP:30 Refill:1 Generic:Y Using:Amoxil Mfg: SmithKline Beecham

▶ **Figure 6-19 Printed encounter note for Howard Cook's follow-up visit.**

Chapter Six Summary

In this chapter you learned to use lists. Lists are selected from the Lists Manager window similar to the way Forms are selected from the Forms Manager window. Both windows are invoked by clicking buttons on the Toolbar.

Lists Lists allow the clinician or medical practice to create a subset of the nomenclature typically used for a particular condition or type of exam. A list usually contains findings in every tab. Because shorter lists mean less scrolling, lists are a sure way to speed the data entry of routine encounters.

A list is accessed by clicking on the button labeled Lists in the Toolbar at the top of the screen and then selecting it from the Lists Manager window.

In this chapter you learned to use the following new buttons on the Toolbar:

List Invokes the Lists Manager window from which you may select and load a List.

Neg The Auto Negative ("Negs") button will automatically set all of the findings that are not already set to "normal" when you are on the Sx or Px tab.

ROS Review of Systems button; toggles on and off. When on (orange) history findings are recorded in the Review of Systems section; when off, history findings are recorded in the History of Present Illness section.

Order Prefaces the highlighted finding with the prefix "ordered" and records the finding in the Plan section of the encounter note. The button is enabled only when a finding is "orderable" but not a medication.

Rx Invokes the Prescription Writer. The button is enabled only if the highlighted finding is a medication.

Task	Exercise	Page
Using the Lists Manager to load a list	33	140
Using the ROS button	33	141
Using the Auto Negative feature	33	144
Recording a medication order using the Prescription Writer (Rx button)	34	149

Testing Your Knowledge of Chapter 6

You may run the Medcin Student Edition software and use your mouse on the screen to answer the following questions:

1. How do you select a list?

2. Name one of the advantages of using a list.

3. What Entry Details field is used with a finding to indicate the patient's fever was "mild"?

Write the meaning of each of the following medical abbreviations as they were used in this chapter.

4. ROS _____

5. HPI _____

6. HEENT _____

7. URI _____

8. Sig _____

9. What is the effect of selecting Sx findings with the ROS button on?

10. What is the effect of selecting Sx findings with the ROS button off?

11. The Auto Negative (Negs) button functions on what two tabs?

12. Which button on the Toolbar invokes the prescription writer?

13. Which section of the SOAP note is a prescription written into?

14. Which section of the encounter note is allergy information written into?

15. You should have produced two narrative documents of patient encounters, which you printed. If you have not already done so, hand these in to your instructor with this test. The printed encounter notes will count as a portion of your grade.

Entering EHR Data Using Forms

Learning Outcomes

After completing this chapter, you should be able to:

- Explain the function of and understand how to use the Forms feature and forms
- Record data using a short intake form
- Use both the Lists and Forms functions in one encounter
- Record prescriptions

The Concept of Forms

In this chapter, we explore the second method of data entry that is used extensively in EHR systems, forms. Electronic forms are one of the easiest ways to use an EHR.

Forms are templates that display a desired group of findings in a consistent position every time. Forms enable quick entry of positive and negative findings, as well as Entry Details field data such as Value or Results.

You already have worked briefly with forms, because the vital signs screen is actually a form. As you have already experienced, vitals are much easier to enter using the Vitals form on which all the necessary findings are arranged with the value fields ready for data entry and the unit of measurement fields preset.

The Vitals form is only a very small example of what can be done with forms. Complete multipage forms can be created that make it fast and easy to document standard types of exams.

Comparison of Lists and Forms

The value of lists is that they are dynamic and expand as necessary. A side effect of this is that sometimes findings do not appear on the screen, because they are in the nonexpanded portion of the tree, or the user must scroll down the list to find them.

Forms, however, are static. Findings have a fixed position on the form and will remain in that location every time the form is used.

Lists arrange findings in the appropriate tab (Sx, Hx, Px, Tx, Dx, and Rx); however, this means that clinicians must change tabs as they work through the encounter. This is not a limitation with forms. The form designer is free to put any finding anywhere on the form. This allows each form to be designed to allow the quickest entry of data for a particular type of encounter. For example, if a medical assistant routinely enters the chief complaint and records the patient's symptoms at the same time she or he takes the vital signs, these could all be placed on one page of the form, even though the findings will appear in three different sections of the note.

Forms offer many additional features to the designer. These include check boxes, drop-down lists, and most of the fields in the Entry Details section. Free-text boxes in a form can be preassigned to a finding; therefore, they do not require the user to locate a free-text finding to record comments.

Note that the forms designer has the option to require entry of data for certain findings before the form can be closed.

Standard Initial Visit Intake for an Adult

The intake form used in the following exercise provides an example of the different looks and features that are possible with forms. These include the unique ability to record two types of history at once, the Auto Negative feature, and other features you will explore during the exercise.

Figure 7-1 is an example of a form that might be found in a medical facility that uses paper medical records. You have probably seen a similar form at your own

Family Practice Medical Center
Anytown, USA

What is the reason you are here today?

_____

Date: _____
Patient Name: _____
Date of Birth: _____
☐ Male ☐ Female

Race: _____

Please check any of the following conditions which you have had

General
☐ Serious Infections
   (e.g. pneumonia)
☐ Diabetes Mellitus
☐ Rheumatic fever
☐ HIV Infection
☐ Cancer

Cardiovascular
☐ High Blood Pressure
☐ Congestive Heart failure
☐ Heart Murmur
☐ Heart Valve Disease
☐ Angina
☐ Heart Attack
☐ High Cholesterol
☐ Abnormal Heart Rhythm
☐ Blood Clot in Veins
☐ Blocked Arteries in Neck
☐ Blocked Arteries in Legs

HEENT
☐ Glaucoma
☐ Allergies "hay fever"
☐ Frequent Ear Infections
☐ Frequent Sinus Infections

Respiratory
☐ Asthma
☐ Emphysema
☐ Blood Colt in Lungs
☐ Sleep Apnea

**Musculoskeletal /
Extremities**
☐ Osteoporosis
☐ Rheumatoid Arthritis
☐ Degenerative Joint Disease
☐ Fibrmyalgia
☐ Neck Pain (herniated disk)
☐ Back Pain (herniated disc)

GI/GU
☐ Stomach Ulcers
☐ Ulcerative Colitis
☐ Crohns Disease
☐ Bleeding from Intestines
☐ Diverticulitis
☐ Colon Polyps
☐ Irritable Bowel Disease
☐ Hepatitis
☐ Cirrhosis of the liver
☐ Liver Failure
☐ Pancreatitis
☐ Gallstones
☐ Kidney Stones
☐ Kidney Failure
☐ Prostate Disease
☐ Endometriosis
☐ Sex Transmitted Infection

Lymphatic / Hematologic
☐ Thyroid Goiter
☐ Over Active Thyroid
☐ Under Active Thyroid
☐ Transfusions
☐ Anemia

Skin / Breast
☐ Acne
☐ Eczema
☐ Psoriasis
☐ Fibrocystic Breast Disease

Neurological / Psychiatric
☐ Chronic Vertigo (Meniere's)
☐ Peripheral Nerve Disease
☐ Migraine Headaches
☐ Stroke
☐ Multiple Sclerosis
☐ Depression
☐ Anxiety

Please check any of the following major illnesses in your family members:

☐ Tuberculosis
☐ Emphysema
☐ Heart Disease
☐ High Blood Pressure
☐ Osteoporosis

☐ Diabetes Mellitus
☐ Thyroid Disease
☐ Anemia
☐ Hemophilia
☐ Other _____

☐ Kidney Disease
☐ Epilepsy
☐ Neurological Disorder
☐ Liver Disease
☐ Other _____

☐ Breast Cancer
☐ Ovarian Cancer
☐ Colon Cancer
☐ Prostate Cancer
☐ Other _____

If you have had surgery please indicate the year:

Year	Surgery	Year	Surgery	Year	Surgery	Year	Surgery
____	Angioplasty	____	Colonoscopy	____	Neurosurgery	____	Tubal ligation
____	Appendectomy	____	Coronary Bypass	____	Sinus Surgery	____	C-Section
____	Back or Neck Surgery	____	Ear Surgery	____	Stomach Surgery	____	Hysterectomy
____	Bladder Surgery	____	Gallbladder	____	Thyroid Surgery	____	Ovary Removed
____	Carotid Artery Surgery	____	Hip Surgery	____	Tonsillectomy	____	Breast Surgery
____	Carpal Tunnel Surgery	____	Inguinal Hernia	____	Trauma Related Surgery	____	Thyroid Surgery
____	Chest/lung Surgery	____	Knee Surgery	____	Vascular Surgery	____	Other

Please indicate when you had the following preventative services:

Date	Immunizations	Date	Tests	Date	Tests / Exams	Date	Tests / Exams
____	Flu Vaccine	____	Chest X-ray	____	Colon Cancer Stool Test	____	Breast Exam
____	Hepatitis Vaccine	____	EKG	____	Flexible Sigmoidoscopy,	____	Mammogram
____	Pneumonia Vaccine	____	Echocardiogram	____	Rectal Exam	____	Pap Smear
____	Tetanus Booster	____	Stress Test	____	Barium Enema	____	Bone Density Test
____	Other	____	Cardiac Angiogram	____	Prostate Cancer Blood Test	____	Date of last Physical Exam

Personal Habits

Tobacco
☐ Never
☐ Previous user
☐ Current user
packs per day _____

Alcohol
☐ Never
☐ Previous user
☐ Current user
drinks per day _____

Caffeine
☐ Never
☐ Previous user
☐ Current user
cups per day _____

Illicit Drugs
☐ Never
☐ Previous user
☐ Current user

▶ Figure 7-1 **Sample intake form from a paper chart.**

doctor's office. As you complete the following exercise, notice the similarities between the paper form and the design of the EHR form.

Guided Exercise 36: Using Forms

In this exercise, you will use an EHR form to record symptoms, history, and a physical exam. In this case, the EHR form has been abridged to shorten the time it takes a student to complete the exercise; a full version of the form as it is used in a medical office would have much more detail. A short intake form might be used by a nurse or medical assistant for prescreening. The clinician would then complete the exam, following up on any abnormal findings.

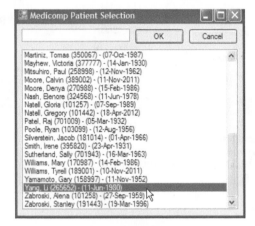

Step 1

If you have not already done so, start the Student Edition software.

Click Select on the Menu bar, and then click Patient.

In the Patient Selection window, locate and click on "Li Yang" as shown in Figure 7-2.

Step 2

Click Select on the Menu bar, and then click New Encounter.

Use the current date and time. Select the reason "Initial Chart Entry Existing Patient" from the drop-down list. Click on the OK button.

Step 3

Enter the chief complaint by locating the button in the Toolbar labeled "Chief" and clicking on it.

In the dialog window that opens, type **Initial patient chart**.

Compare your screen to Figure 7-3 before clicking on the button labeled "Close the note form."

Step 4

Click on the Forms button in the Toolbar at the top of the screen.

In the Forms Manager window, select the form labeled "Short Intake," as shown in Figure 7-4. The Short Intake form shown in Figure 7-5 will be displayed.

Step 5

Compare your screen to Figure 7-5. Take a few minutes to study the form on your screen.

▶ Figure 7-2 **Selecting Li Yang from the Patient Selection window.**

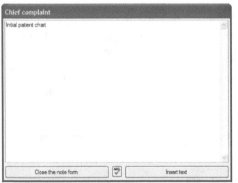

▶ Figure 7-3 **Chief complaint dialog for initial patient chart.**

Note that at the top of the form there are tabs labeled Review of Systems, Medical History, Physical Examination, and Outline View. This form has three pages on which you may enter data. In subsequent steps, you will use each of these pages to explore the features of this form.

Probably the first thing you noticed are columns of check boxes with Y and N next to them. This is very similar to a paper form and very intuitive. With almost no training, people understand Y means "yes" and N means "no."

► **Figure 7-4 Select Short Intake in the Forms Manager window.**

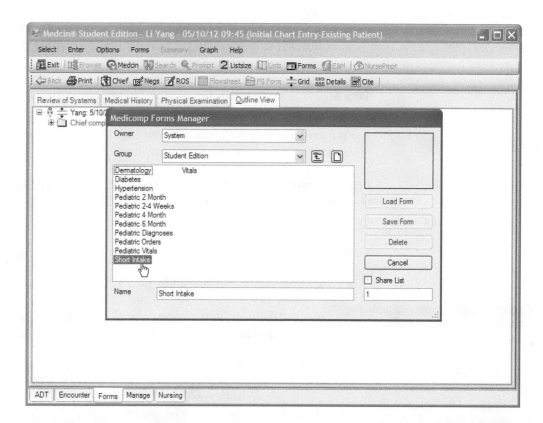

► **Figure 7-5 Review of Symptoms tab of Short Intake form.**

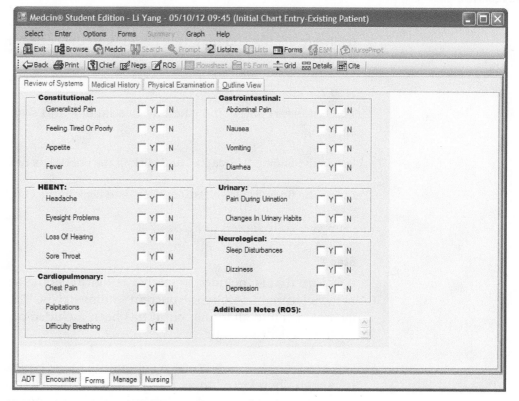

Check boxes work very simply. Here is how:

✓ If you click your mouse on an empty box, a check mark appears. The finding will be recorded in the patient's record.

✓ If you change your mind and click in the opposite box, the check mark moves to the box you just clicked.

✓ If you didn't want either box checked, click on whichever box already has the check mark and you will be asked to confirm that you want the finding removed (as shown in Figure 7-6).

Step 6

On the Review of Symptoms tab, if you put a check in the Y box, it means that the patient has that symptom. If you put a check in the N box, this means that the patient does not have that symptom.

Practice using the check boxes with the finding Headache, which is located in the section of the form labeled "HEENT." Remember, HEENT stands for head, eyes, ears, nose, and throat.

Locate the finding "Headache" and click in the check box next to the letter "Y."

Now click the mouse in the check box next to the letter "N." Did the check mark move?

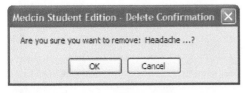

▶ Figure 7-6 **Confirmation that you want to remove a finding.**

Although you cannot see the encounter note at this moment, you just changed the note from "Headache" to "No headache."

Click the mouse again in the same box that already has the check mark in it; this should be next to the letter "N." The confirmation message shown in Figure 7-6 should appear. Click on the OK button. Both check boxes should now be empty.

Remember, even though the form looks different than the Encounter tab, you really are adding and removing findings on the patient note when you work with the form.

Step 7

The patient reports that she has headaches and some nights has trouble sleeping.

Locate the finding "Headache" and click in the check box next to the letter "Y."

Locate the finding "Sleep Disturbances" and click in the check box next to the letter "Y."

Compare your screen to Figure 7-7.

Step 8

A feature that is included in many EHR forms is the ability to see where in the nomenclature hierarchy the current finding exists. This feature is not necessarily designed into all forms, but it has been included on the Short Intake form for the Student Edition.

Left and Right Mouse Buttons A computer mouse typically has at least two buttons, usually referred to as the "left-click" and "right-click" buttons. In this step you will use the right-click button. If your mouse has only one button, use the Alternate Instructions for Left Mouse Button provided in the accompanying box.

Position the mouse pointer over the word "Headache" (not over the Y/N check boxes.) The finding will become highlighted in white and the mouse pointer will change shape to include a question mark. When your mouse pointer

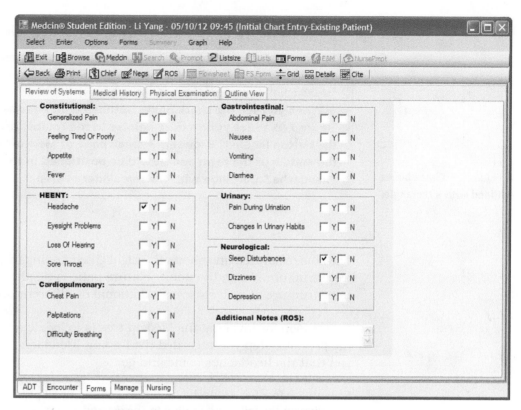

▶ Figure 7-7 **Recording Headache and Sleep Disturbances.**

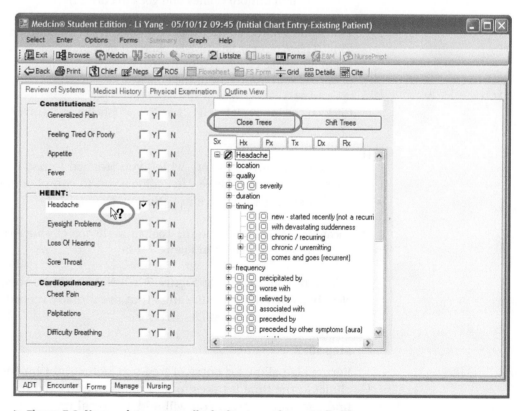

▶ Figure 7-8 **Nomenclature pane displaying tree of current finding.**

looks like the one circled in red in Figure 7-8, click the **right-click button** on your mouse. A small pane of Medcin findings will open in the middle of the form.

Alternate Instructions for Left Mouse Button

An alternative to using the right mouse button to open the nomenclature pane in a form is to click the left button of your mouse on the finding name "Headache" (not over the Y/N check boxes).

When you see the check boxes outlined with a rectangle (as shown in Figure 7-9), move your mouse pointer to the Toolbar and locate and click on the button labeled "Browse." A small pane of Medcin findings will open in the middle of the form and should be positioned in the tree on the finding "Headache." Continue with the remainder of step 8.

Headache ☑ Y ☐ N

▶ Figure 7-9 **Check boxes outlined with a rectangle.**

The nomenclature pane shows the highlighted finding in the context of the Medcin tree structure. When the nomenclature pane is displayed, you can expand the tree structure as well as select additional or different findings.

One reason for invoking the Medcin tree is to locate a more specific finding. In the previous step you recorded the finding "Headache," but the patient informs you that the headaches come and go.

Expand the tree for Headache by clicking on the small plus sign next to "timing." Locate and click on the following finding in the expanded tree:

● (red button) Comes and goes (recurrent)

Two buttons at the top of the pane allow you to close or reposition it. The button labeled "Shift Trees" moves the browser pane left or right so you can see a part of the form that might otherwise be covered by the pane. The button labeled "Close Trees" closes the pane to restore your view of the entire form.

Click on the button labeled "Close Trees" (shown in Figure 7-8 circled in red).

Step 9

The Auto Negative button, which you learned to use in Exercise 33, also can be enabled in forms. This feature allows you to complete form pages quickly whenever most of the answers are "No" or "Normal."

Locate the "Negs" button in the Toolbar at the top of your form. Click your mouse on the Negs button (highlighted in Figure 7-10).

Compare your screen to Figure 7-10. Note what happened. Note that Auto Negative does not alter findings that are already recorded, as in this example, "Headache" and "Sleep Disturbances."

Step 10

Forms also allow for entry of free-text notes right on the form. This saves the clinician the time it takes to add notes to entry details or to open free-text findings. In this step, you will add a clinical impression to the ROS findings.

In the box at the bottom of your screen labeled "Additional Notes (ROS)," type the following text: **Patient denies depression but seems very sad.**

Compare your screen to Figure 7-11 before proceeding.

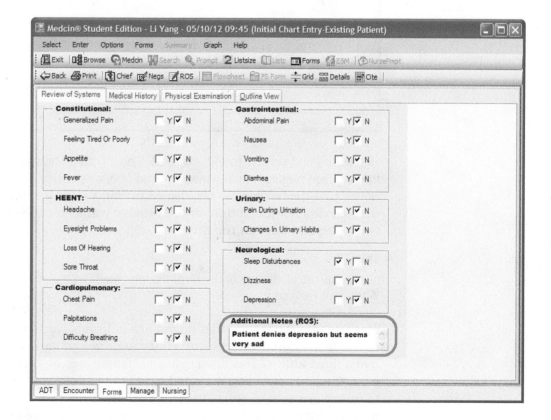

Step 11

During the course of this exercise, you have been recording findings in the encounter note with every click of your mouse on the form, but you cannot see them as you can on the Encounter tab.

In Forms, the Outline View tab allows you to take a quick look at the findings you have selected for the encounter note. Before entering data in the rest of the form, take a moment to look at what has been entered so far.

Locate and click on the tab labeled "Outline View" at the top of your form (circled in red in Figure 7-12).

Click the small plus signs next to the folder icons to expand them to show the findings.

▶ Figure 7-12 **Outline View.**

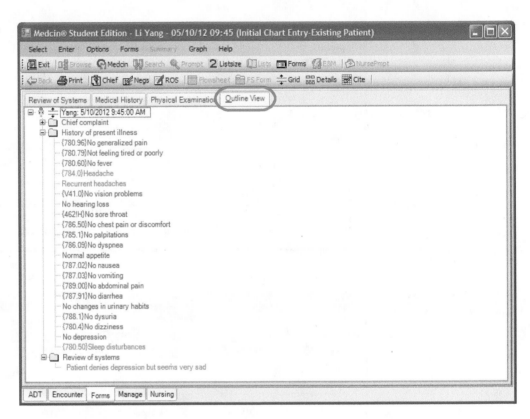

Compare your screen to Figure 7-12. The Outline View uses blue text when the findings are negative or normal and red text when they are positive or abnormal. Notice that the headaches are also recurrent; this is the finding you entered from the tree view. At the bottom of the window you also can see in red text the free-text note you added in the previous step.

Step 12

Locate the tab at the top of the form labeled "Medical History" (circled in red in Figure 7-13), and click on it.

This page illustrates another advantage of forms. Normally, when you do an intake history on a patient, you go through many items twice: "Have you ever had a heart attack? Has anyone in your family ever had a heart attack?" On this page, the form has been designed to save the clinician time by making it easy to record answers to either personal, family history, or both types of questions in two columns. Compare the information on this tab of the EHR form with the paper form in Figure 7-1.

Step 13

Sometimes patients do not know the medical history of other family members; therefore, you will only record findings the patient is sure about. As the medical

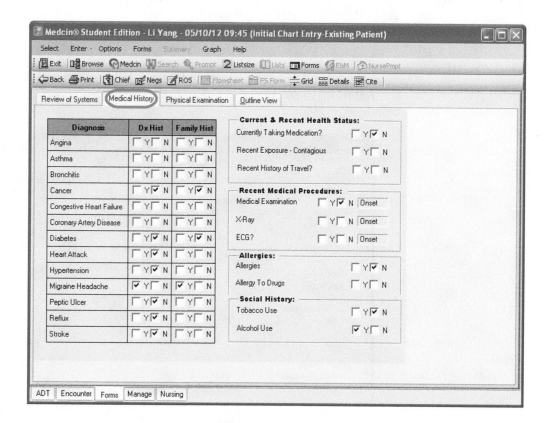

► **Figure 7-13 Medical History page of Short Intake form.**

assistant asks Ms. Yang the history questions, the patient will only know the answer to some of them.

Enter the Dx History and Family History only for the following items:

Diagnosis	Dx Hist	Family Hist
Cancer	✓ N	✓ N
Diabetes	✓ N	✓ N
Heart Attack	✓ N	
Hypertension	✓ N	
Migraine	✓ Y	✓ Y
Peptic Ulcer	✓ N	
Reflux	✓ N	
Stroke	✓ N	

Complete the rest of her medical history in the right side of the form by locating and clicking on the check boxes as follows:

Currently Taking Medication?	✓ N
Recent Medical Examination	✓ N
Allergies	✓ N
Tobacco Use	✓ N
Alcohol Use	✓ Y

Carefully compare your screen to Figure 7-13 before proceeding.

Step 14

Locate the tab at the top of the form labeled "Physical Examination" (circled in red in Figure 7-14), and click on it.

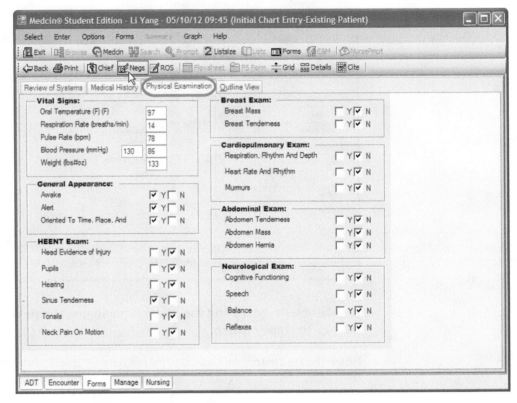

▶ Figure 7-14 **Physical Exam page of Short Intake form.**

The first thing you will notice about this page is that it includes a place to record vital signs in the upper left corner of the page. Recording vital signs as part of the intake physical saves the time it would take to load the Vitals form separately. This page illustrates how forms can combine many different elements to make data entry more convenient.

Enter the following vital signs for Li Yang:

Temperature:	**97**
Respiration:	**14**
Pulse:	**78**
BP:	**130/86**
Weight:	**133**

Step 15

During the exam, the clinician observes sinus tenderness. Locate the finding "Sinus Tenderness" and click the check box for "Y."

Everything else is normal. Click on the button labeled "Negs" on the Toolbar at the top of your screen (highlighted in Figure 7-14).

Remember you can use the button to quickly document "normals" on Symptoms and Physical Exam findings.

Compare your screen to Figure 7-14.

Did you see that the findings in the General Appearance group were checked Y instead of N by the Auto Negative feature? That is because for some findings such as these, the normal state is to be awake, alert, and oriented. If these were checked No, the condition would be abnormal. The Auto Negative feature is really an Auto Normal feature.

Step 16

Click on the Encounter tab at the bottom of your screen to view the full text of the encounter note that was completed from within the form.

Click on the Dx tab in the left pane and enter an assessment.

Locate and click the red button for the following finding:

- (red button) Normal examination

Compare your screen to Figure 7-15. Scroll the right pane so that you can view the entire contents of the note.

► Figure 7-15 **Encounter note entered using a form.**

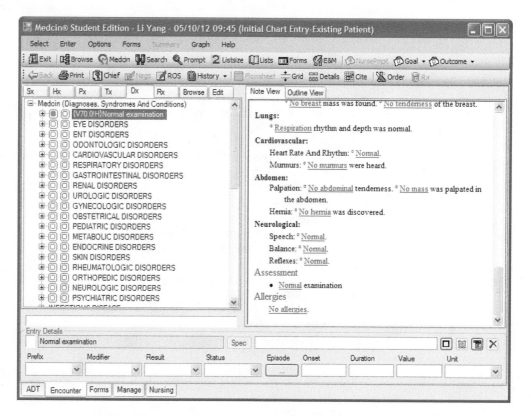

Step 17

This exercise was intended to demonstrate how forms can be used to speed through pages of routine questions and provide the convenience of free-text or Entry Details fields as part of the form. Although the exercise does not create a medically complete intake history and a physical, you have successfully completed the goals of this exercise.

Step 18

Click on the Print button on the Toolbar at the top of your screen to invoke the Print Data window.

Be certain there is a check mark in the box next to "Current Encounter" and then click on the appropriate button to either print or export a file, as directed by your instructor.

Compare your printout or file output to Figure 7-16. If it is correct, hand it in to your instructor. If there are any differences (other than the date or patient's age), review the previous steps in the exercise and find your error.

(Note your computer will print out two pages; however, the page breaks may not be in the same place as Figure 7-16. The page breaks vary by the type of printer and will not affect your grade.)

Li Yang   Page 1 of 2

Student: *your name or ID here*
Patient: Li Yang: F: 6/11/1980: 5/10/2012 09:45 AM
Chief complaint
The Chief Complaint is: Initial patient chart.
History of present illness
        Li Yang is a 31 year old female.
        She reported: Headache recurrent.
        No depression. Sleep disturbances.
        No generalized pain, not feeling tired or poorly, and no fever. No vision problems. No hearing loss and no sore throat. No chest pain or discomfort and no palpitations. No dyspnea. Normal appetite, no nausea, no vomiting, no abdominal pain, and no diarrhea. No changes in urinary habits and no dysuria. No dizziness.
Past medical/surgical history
Reported History:
        Medical: No recent medical examination.
        Medications: Not taking medication.
Diagnosis History:
        No acute myocardial infarction.
        No hypertension.
        No esophageal reflux
        No peptic ulcer.
        No diabetes mellitus.
        Migraine headache.
        No stroke syndrome.
        No cancer
Personal history
Behavioral: No tobacco use.
Alcohol: Alcohol use.

Continued on the following page...

▶ **Figure 7-16a** **Printout of encounter note for Li Yang (page 1 of 2).**

Family history
    No diabetes mellitus
    Migraine headache
    No cancer.
Review of systems
Patient denies depression but seems very sad.
Physical findings
Vital Signs:

Vital Signs/Measurements	Value	Normal Range
Oral temperature	97 F	97.6 - 99.6
RR	14 breaths/min	18 - 26
PR	78 bpm	50 - 100
Blood pressure	130/86 mmHg	100-120/56-80
Weight	133 lbs	98 - 183

General Appearance:
    ° Awake. ° Alert. ° Oriented to time, place, and person.
Head:
    Injuries: ° No evidence of a head injury.
Neck:
    Maneuvers: ° Neck pain was not elicited by motion.
Eyes:
    General/bilateral:
      Pupils: ° Normal.
Ears:
    General/bilateral:
      Hearing: ° No hearing abnormalities.
Nose:
    General/bilateral:
      Sinus Tenderness: • Tenderness of sinuses.
Pharynx:
    Oropharynx: ° Tonsils showed no abnormalities.
Breasts:
    General/bilateral:
      ° No breast mass was found. ° No tenderness of the breast.
Lungs:
    ° Respiration rhythm and depth was normal.
Cardiovascular:
    Heart Rate and Rhythm: ° Normal.
    Murmurs: ° No murmurs were heard.
Abdomen:
    Palpation: ° No abdominal tenderness. ° No mass was palpated in the abdomen.
    Hernia: ° No hernia was discovered.
Neurological:
    ° Cognitive functioning was normal.
    Speech: ° Normal.
    Balance: ° Normal.
    Reflexes: ° Normal.
Allergies
    No allergies.

▶ **Figure 7-16b Printout of encounter note for Li Yang (page 2 of 2).**

Customized Forms

Forms are not limited to the pages used in this exercise. The Forms feature also allows you to organize questions in the order you would ask them, regardless of where the findings may be grouped in the Medcin nomenclature hierarchy.

Forms can be designed to include pages for any of the findings expected to be needed for a particular type of visit. For example, a therapy page is an excellent means of having quick access to standard treatments for specific conditions. Medical facilities that have a large number of forms customized to their style of practice succeed very well in implementing an EHR. Form design tools are a part of almost every EHR system on the market.

Critical Thinking Exercise 37: Using a Form and a List

In this exercise you will use both the form and the list from the previous exercises. Patient John Lewis, who was seen previously for acute sinusitis, has returned for a follow-up visit.

Patient John Lewis has been experiencing stuffy sinus pain. The medical office has scheduled a brief office visit for him to see the nurse practitioner. Using what you have learned so far, document Mr. Lewis's brief encounter.

Step 1

If you have not already done so, start the Student Edition software.

Click Select on the Menu bar, and then click Patient.

In the Patient Selection window, locate and click on "John Lewis."

Step 2

The patient was previously seen and diagnosed with acute sinusitis. The patient is returning for a follow-up visit.

Click Select on the Menu bar, and then click New Encounter.

Select the reason "Follow-up" from the drop-down list.

Make sure you have selected the reason correctly. You may use the current date for this exercise.

Step 3

Enter the chief complaint by locating the button in the Toolbar labeled "Chief" and clicking on it.

In the dialog window that opens, type **Sinusitis follow-up**.

Click on the button labeled "Close the note form."

Step 4

Click on the Forms button in the Toolbar at the top of the screen.

In the Forms Manager window, select the Form labeled "Short Intake."

Step 5

On the Review of Symptoms tab, locate the section of the form labeled "HEENT."

Locate the finding Headache and click in the check box next to the letter "Y."

Step 6

Position the mouse pointer over the word "Headache" (not over the Y/N check boxes.)

The finding will become highlighted in white and the mouse pointer will change shape to include a question mark. Click the **right-click button** on your mouse. A small pane of Medcin findings will open in the middle of the form.

Step 7

When the nomenclature pane is displayed, expand the tree by clicking on the small plus sign next to "Location."

Locate and click on the following finding in the Medcin tree currently displayed in your form:

● (red button) Headache in the forehead (Frontal)

Click on the button labeled "Close Trees."

Step 8

Locate and click on the "ROS" button in the Toolbar at the top of your form.

Verify the button is orange.

Locate and click on the "Negs" button in the Toolbar at the top of your form.

Locate and click on the "ROS" button in the Toolbar at the top of your form. Verify the button is blue.

All items on the Review of Symptoms tab should now have a check in either the Y or N boxes.

Step 9

Locate the tab at the top of the form labeled "Medical History."

Locate the finding "Currently Taking Medication" and click in the check box next to the letter "Y."

Position the mouse pointer over the finding "Currently Taking Medication" (not over the Y/N check boxes) and click the **right-click button** on your mouse.

Scroll the list of Medcin findings that opened on the left of the form downward to locate and click on the following finding:

● (red button) over-the-counter

Click on the button labeled "Close Trees" at the top of the pane.

Step 10

Locate the finding Allergies and click in the check box next to the letter "N."

Step 11

Locate the tab at the top of the form labeled "Physical Examination."

Enter Mr. Lewis's vital signs in the corresponding fields as follows:

Temperature: **99.7**

Respiration: **17**

Pulse: **68**

BP: **120/88**

Weight: **177**

Step 12

Locate the finding "Sinus Tenderness" (in the HEENT section) and click in the check box next to the letter "Y."

Locate and click on the "Negs" button in the Toolbar at the top of your form.

All items on the Physical Examination tab should now have data.

Step 13

Locate and click on the Encounter tab at the bottom of your screen to return to the encounter view.

Locate and click on the Lists button in the Toolbar at the top of your screen. The Lists Manager window will be invoked.

Locate and highlight the list named Adult URI. Click your mouse on the button labeled "Load List."

Step 14

If you are not on the Sx tab, click on it. Verify that the first line of the Medcin Nomenclature in the left pane reads: "Templates (Symptoms)."

Locate and click on the following symptom findings:

- (red button) Fever
- (red button) Sinus pain
- (red button) Nasal discharge
- (red button) Nasal blockage (from stuffiness)

Locate and click on the "Negs" button in the Toolbar at the top of your screen.

Step 15

Click on the Hx tab. Locate and click on the following History findings:

- (red button) Recent upper respiratory infection (URI)

Locate and click on the red button next to the following finding:

- (red button) current smoker

In the Value field at the bottom of your screen type the number **20**.

Step 16

Click on the Px tab to document the physical exam.

Locate and click on the following Physical Exam findings.

- (red button) Nasal Discharge
- (red button) Nasal Discharge Purulent

Locate and click on the "Negs" button in the Toolbar at the top of your screen.

Step 17

Click on the Dx tab and then locate and click on the following finding:

- (red button) Sinusitis Acute

Step 18

Click on the Rx tab and then locate and click on the following finding:

- (red button) Fluids

Step 19

Locate and highlight the finding "Antibacterial Amoxicillin."

Locate and click on the button labeled Rx on the Toolbar. The prescription writing window will be invoked.

Step 20

Locate and click your mouse on the Sig: "500 milligram cap 1 po q8h 10 DSP:30."

The next window displaying available brands (see Figure 6-15 in Chapter 6) will be displayed automatically.

Step 21

Locate and click on "Amoxil SmithKline Beecham."

! **Alert**

Do not close or exit the encounter until you have a printed copy in your hand. *You will lose your work if you exit before printing.*

Step 22

Locate the "Generic Allowed" fields. Click in the small circle next to "Yes." The small circle is then filled in.

Click on the button labeled "Save Rx."

Step 23

Click on the Print button on the Toolbar at the top of your screen to invoke the Print Data window.

Be certain there is a check mark in the box next to "Current Encounter" and then click on the appropriate button to either print or export a file, as directed by your instructor.

Compare your printout or file output to Figure 7-17. If it is correct, hand it in to your instructor. If there are any differences (other than the date or patient's age), review the previous steps in the exercise and find your error.

(Note your computer will print out two pages; however, the page breaks may not be in the same place as Figure 7-17. The page breaks vary by the type of printer and will not affect your grade.)

Student: *your name or ID here*
Patient: John Lewis: M: 5/05/1979: 5/10/2012 02:30 PM
Chief complaint
The Chief Complaint is: Sinusitis follow-up.
History of present illness
    John Lewis is a 33 year old male.
    He reported: Fever. No chills.
    Headache frontal and sinus pain.
    No earache and no discharge from the ears. Nasal discharge and nasal passage blockage.
    No swollen glands in the neck. No cough, not coughing up sputum, and no hemoptysis.
    No muscle aches.
Past medical/surgical history
Reported History:
    Medical: A recent URI.
    Medications: Taking over-the-counter medications.
Personal history
    Behavioral: Current smoker was 20 years.
Review of systems
    Systemic: No generalized pain and not feeling tired or poorly.
    Eyes: No vision problems.
    Otolaryngeal: No hearing loss and no sore throat.
    Cardiovascular: No chest pain or discomfort and no palpitations.
    Pulmonary: No dyspnea.
    Gastrointestinal: Normal appetite, no nausea, no vomiting, no abdominal pain, and no diarrhea.
    Genitourinary: No changes in urinary habits and no dysuria.
    Neurological: No dizziness.
    Psychological: No depression and no sleep disturbances.
Physical findings
Vital Signs:

Vital Signs/Measurements	Value	Normal Range
Oral temperature	99.7 F	97.6 - 99.6
RR	17 breaths/min	18 - 26
PR	68 bpm	50 - 100
Blood pressure	120/88 mmHg	100-120/60-80
Weight	177 lbs	125 - 225

General Appearance:
    ° Awake. ° Alert. ° Oriented to time, place, and person.
Head:
    Injuries: ° No evidence of a head injury.
Neck:
    Maneuvers: ° Neck pain was not elicited by motion.
Eyes:
    General/bilateral:
      Pupils: ° Normal.
Ears:
    General/bilateral:
      Hearing: ° No hearing abnormalities.
Nose:
    General/bilateral:
      Discharge: • Nasal discharge seen. • Purulent nasal discharge.
      Cavity: ° Nasal septum normal. ° Nasal turbinate not swollen.
      Sinus Tenderness: • Tenderness of sinuses.

Continued on the following page...

▶ **Figure 7-17a Printed encounter note for John Lewis's follow-up visit (page 1 of 2).**

Pharynx:
Oropharynx: ° Tonsils showed no abnormalities.
Mucosal: ° Pharynx was not inflamed.

Lymph Nodes:
° Normal.

Breasts:
General/bilateral:
° No breast mass was found. ° No tenderness of the breast.

Lungs:
° Respiration rhythm and depth was normal. ° Respiratory movements were normal. ° Chest was normal to percussion. ° No wheezing was heard. ° No rhonchi were heard. ° No rales/crackles were heard.

Cardiovascular:
Heart Rate and Rhythm: ° Normal.
Murmurs: ° No murmurs were heard.

Abdomen:
Palpation: ° No abdominal tenderness. ° No mass was palpated in the abdomen.
Hernia: ° No hernia was discovered.

Neurological:
° Cognitive functioning was normal.
Speech: ° Normal.
Balance: ° Normal.
Reflexes: ° Normal.

Assessment
• Acute sinusitis

Allergies
No allergies.

Plan
• Fluids
• Amoxicillin
500 mg cap (1 po q8h 10) DISP:30 Refill:1 Generic:Y Using:Amoxil Mfg: SmithKline Beecham

▶ Figure 7-17b **Printed encounter note for John Lewis's follow-up visit (page 2 of 2).**

Chapter Seven Summary

In this chapter you learned that Forms can be used to enter various types of data. Forms display a desired group of findings in a presentation that allows for quick entry of not only positive and negative findings but of any Entry Details fields such as Value or Results as well.

Forms also provide other features that lists cannot:

◆ Forms are static; findings have a fixed position on forms, and will consistently remain in that position, every time the form is used.

◆ Findings from multiple sections of the nomenclature can be mixed on the same page of the form in any way that will enable the quickest data entry.

◆ Forms may include check boxes, drop-down lists, the fields in the Entry Details section, the onset date, and free-text boxes to record comments.

◆ Forms can control which findings are required and which are optional; every question on a Form does not have to be answered for every visit.

A form is accessed by clicking on the Forms button on the Toolbar, and then selecting the desired form from the Forms Manager window.

The Outline View allows you to see the findings that have been selected without leaving the Forms tab.

Testing Your Knowledge of Chapter 7

You may run the Medcin Student Edition software and use your mouse on the screen to answer the following questions:

1. How do you select forms?

2. List three features forms have that lists do not.

3. What is the purpose of the Outline View Tab on a Form?

4. What is the advantage of entering the patient's medical history and family history on a form?

5. Why are family history items sometimes left unanswered?

6. How do you access the nomenclature without closing a form?

7. How do you close the nomenclature pane when it is opened on a form?

8. Which button on the Toolbar sets findings that have not been otherwise selected to normal?

9. What was the diagnosis for John Lewis?

Circle True or False for the following statements:

10. Findings from multiple sections of the nomenclature can be mixed on the same page of the form.

    True   False

11. The ROS and Negs buttons are inactive while using a Form.

    True   False

12. A list and a form cannot be used on the same encounter note.

    True   False

13. Clicking a check box more than once on a form will create duplicate findings in the note.

    True   False

14. The Outline View displays blue text when the findings are negative or normal and red text when they are positive or abnormal.

    True   False

15. You should have produced two narrative documents of patient encounters, which you printed. If you have not already done so, hand these in to your instructor with this test. The printed encounter notes will count as a portion of your grade.

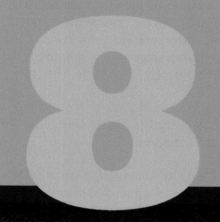

EHR Coding and Reimbursement

Learning Outcomes

After completing this chapter, you should be able to:

◆ Explain why billing codes are important in an EHR system

◆ Show how Evaluation and Management (E&M) codes are determined

◆ Name and describe key components of E&M codes

◆ Read and understand the tables used in CMS guidelines

◆ Explain how the level of key components determines the level of the E&M code

◆ Use E&M Calculator software

◆ Correctly use and document the Time factor to change the level of an E&M code

The EHR and Reimbursement

There is no question that healthcare providers must be paid for their services and that the vast majority of those payments are from insurance plans, which require the use of standard codes. Some clinical workers ignore or resist a discussion of the relationship of the EHR to reimbursement, considering it the responsibility of the "billing" department. Unfortunately, that is not the case.

Whether the clinician is a doctor, nurse, or medical assistant, how and what that person documents in the patient chart has everything to do with what the medical facility is going to be paid for treating the patient.

Insurance plan audits follow this dictum: *If it isn't documented, it wasn't done.* This means that no matter how long the medical assistant and patient discussed the patient's history and symptoms, no matter how thoroughly the medical assistant or nurse assessed the patient, no matter how brilliant the doctor's diagnosis, if those findings aren't documented with sufficient detail in the chart, the auditor will assume that those portions of the exam were never performed.

Knowing there is a direct relationship between the completeness of your clinical documentation and the financial well-being of your medical facility can help you understand the necessity of this chapter. If your interest is primarily clinical and not administrative, have no fear of this chapter. It is not intended to train you as a medical coder or billing specialist. A complete medical coding course could not be taught in one chapter anyway.

The purpose of this chapter is to help you understand the guidelines used for calculating reimbursement by analyzing an encounter recorded in an EHR.

The EHR Helps Meet Government Mandates

The U.S. government, Medicare, and insurance regulations financially affect all healthcare facilities. Adoption of an EHR system can not only improve patient care, as described in earlier chapters, but can also ensure reimbursement for services provided. In this chapter we are going to discuss three factors affected by an EHR:

1. Incentives and penalties
2. Proper coding of diagnoses
3. Factors of evaluation and management.

Incentives and Penalties

In Chapter 1 we discussed the Health Information Technology for Economic and Clinical Health (HITECH) Act.[1] The government firmly believes in the benefits of using electronic health records. It is encouraging the widespread adoption of EHR by authorizing Medicare to make incentive payments to doctors and hospitals that use a certified EHR. This means that a practice adopting an EHR actually gets paid more than a practice continuing to use paper charts. Providers that

---

[1]H.R. 1 American Recovery and Reinvestment Act of 2009, Title XIII Health Information Technology for Economic and Clinical Health, February 17, 2009.

implement and use a certified EHR in a meaningful way prior to 2015 are eligible for incentives. Here are some of the "meaningful use" requirements:

◆ Use a certified EHR.

◆ Submit most prescriptions electronically.

◆ Report clinical quality measures.

◆ Use an EHR that interconnects electronically for healthcare delivery.

◆ Report billing codes indicating that patient encounters were recorded using an EHR.

After 2015 Medicare will begin to administer financial penalties for physicians and hospitals that do not use an EHR. These will involve reducing the provider's payments by 1% per year for up to five years. By 2020 a provider still using paper charts will have payments reduced by 5%.

HIPAA-Required Code Sets

HIPAA[2] law regulates many things, including the privacy and security of health records. It also standardized healthcare transactions and required the use of the ICD-9-CM, CPT-4, and HCPCS code sets.

ICD-9-CM Diagnosis Codes

ICD-9-CM stands for International Classification of Diseases, ninth revision, with clinical modifications. It is a system of standardized codes developed collaboratively among the World Health Organization (WHO) and 10 international centers. Each of the encounters you have documented in the previous exercises included an assessment finding that was selected on the Dx tab of the software. As you are already aware, Dx is an acronym for "diagnosis." Diagnoses are assigned codes using the ICD-9-CM code set. (*Note:* The United States is scheduled to move to a newer version, ICD-10, in October 2013.)

The ICD-9-CM codes are used to classify causes of mortality and disease conditions into statistical, reportable data. ICD-9-CM codes are also used daily by clinicians and medical billing departments because they are required for insurance claims.

◆ Reimbursement for most inpatient hospitals is based entirely on the diagnosis-related group (DRG) determined from the primary and secondary diagnoses assigned by the attending physician.

◆ For both inpatient and outpatient facilities, the use of the correct ICD-9-CM code on a claim serves to explain or justify the medical reason for the services being billed.

◆ Outpatient billing requires one or more ICD-9-CM codes to be assigned to every procedure. Furthermore the diagnosis must correspond to the procedure. For example, you can't bill for an eye exam using the diagnosis for a broken toe.

---

[2]Health Insurance Portability and Accountability Act, Administrative Simplification Subsection, Title 2, subsection f.

Where paper charts are used, the diagnosis is often indicated by circling a code on a preprinted form called an encounter form. However, the preprinted codes on the form may not be as specific as the clinician's assessment. The clinician must also be careful to use the same terminology in the dictation as the ICD-9-CM description, or the billing for the visit may not match the transcribed encounter note.

When an EHR is used, a "cross-walk" or internal reference table assigns the ICD-9-CM codes automatically based on the clinician's assessment finding(s). You can see an example of this in the Student Edition Outline View pane shown in Figure 8-1.

▶ **Figure 8-1 ICD-9-CM codes displayed in Outline View tab.**

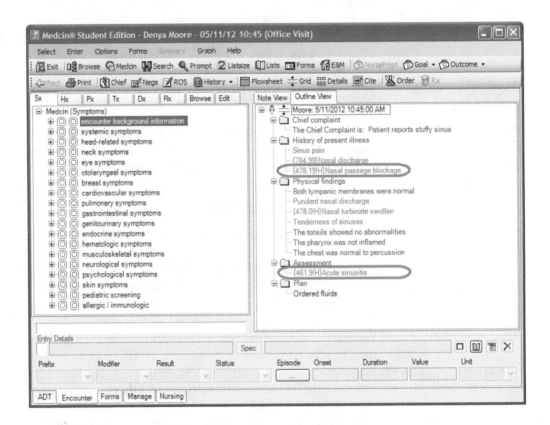

The advantage of using an EHR with a codified nomenclature is that the codes billed will always be in sync with the note that is produced.

CPT-4 and HCPCS Codes

In addition to standard codes for diagnoses, HIPAA requires the use of CPT-4 and HCPCS codes for procedures. CPT stands for Current Procedural Terminology, fourth edition. It was developed and is maintained by the American Medical Association (AMA). HCPCS stands for Healthcare Common Procedure Coding System. It was developed by the CMS to code for supplies, injectable medications, and blood products. CPT-4 is incorporated into the HCPCS standard even though it is separately maintained by the AMA.

Evaluation and Management (E&M) Codes

While some CPT-4 codes represent a specific medical procedure, the most frequently used portion of the CPT-4 code set is the Evaluation and Management

(E&M) codes. These CPT-4 codes are used to bill for nearly every kind of patient encounter, including physician office visits, inpatient hospital exams, nursing home visits, consults, emergency room (ER) doctors, and scores of other services. E&M codes are used by virtually all specialties.

At one time E&M billing was based on the provider's judgment of how complex the visit was. However, Medicare has developed strict guidelines for determining how the level of exam justified the level of E&M code. The time spent with the patient is no longer the controlling factor.

E&M guidelines were first published in 1995 and revamped in 1997.[3] They determine the CPT-4 E&M code based almost exclusively on the findings documented in the encounter note. Gone are the days when a physician might perform a very adequate physical but scribble only a few lines in the chart.

Four Levels of E&M Codes

There are four levels of E&M codes for each type of visit. The levels range from the least complicated exam (level 1) to the most complex exam (level 4). The level is important because a provider's "allowed payment" amount is proportionate to the level of the exam (with level 1 paying the least, and level 4 paying the most).

Where the service is rendered is an important consideration as well. There are separate categories of E&M codes for different locations such as office visits, inpatient exams, ER exams, and so on. Each category of E&M codes has at least four codes representing the four levels of service. Some categories have more than four E&M codes because there are subcategories, for example, new patient versus established patient. The exercises in this chapter use the E&M codes for office visits.

How the Level of an E&M Code Is Determined

Seven components are evaluated to determine the level of E&M services:

- History
- Examination
- Medical decision making
- Counseling
- Coordination of care
- Nature of presenting problem
- Time.

Three components—*history, examination,* and *medical decision making*—are the key components in determining the level of E&M services. The level of each key component is determined separately. The level of E&M code is derived from the highest level of two or three key components. There is one exception. For services such as psychiatry, which consist predominantly of counseling or coordination of care, time is the key or controlling factor determining the level of E&M service.

---

[3]Providers are permitted to use either guideline. Examples in this book use the 1997 guideline.

This chapter explains each of the components, the levels within the key components, and how they are combined to calculate the E&M code. A later exercise will also show how time can become an overriding factor, justifying a higher level code for visits that require more time for counseling the patient.

Undercoding

In an office using paper charts, clinicians often select the E&M code by circling a code on a paper encounter form. These clinicians are at risk. If they select a code that is at a higher level than the dictated note supports, they can be fined. To avoid risk, many practices *undercode* (choosing a code one level below what they believe to be correct), taking the attitude "better safe than sorry." This is bad for the practice financially; they are losing payment for their work. When clinicians undercode by one level, it is the same as seeing 80 patients and getting paid for seeing 60.

Accurate Coding

The clinician using an EHR doesn't worry about the mandate "*If it isn't documented, it wasn't done*" because it is *always* documented. EHR systems that use standardized nomenclatures have a codified record of the encounter. This enables the software to use data in the encounter note to calculate the correct E&M code for billing.

EHR systems analyze the amount and type of data and accurately determine the correct E&M code at the correct level. Many EHR systems can show the provider how the calculation was determined, thus giving the provider confidence that the code can be substantiated. In addition to E&M codes, the EHR can suggest CPT-4 codes for other procedures performed during the encounter.

When the EHR is an integrated component of practice management software, or when it is interfaced to a practice management system, the ICD-9-CM, CPT-4, and HCPCS codes can transfer directly to the billing or charge posting module. Most practice management systems do not post the charges automatically, but transfer them as "pending" charges. The charges are reviewed by a billing or coding specialist before being "posted" to the patient's account or billed to insurance.

Using EHR Software to Understand E&M Codes

In the next few exercises, we are going to focus on understanding E&M codes. The Student Edition software contains an E&M code calculator. You are going to use that tool while learning how E&M codes are derived.

Guided Exercise 38: Calculating the E&M Code from an Exam

In this exercise, you are going to learn how to use the E&M Calculator by using a previously stored encounter that is already in your system. Using a previous encounter will allow you to focus on understanding the E&M codes themselves without worrying about creating the note.

Step 1

If you have not already done so, start the Student Edition software.

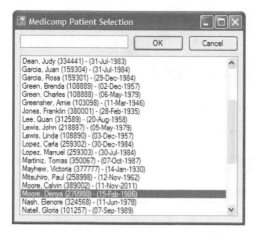

Figure 8-2 Select patient Denya Moore.

Click Select on the Menu bar, and then click Patient.

In the Patient Selection window, locate and click on "Denya Moore" (as shown in Figure 8-2).

Step 2

Click Select on the Menu bar, and then click "Existing Encounter." This is a new feature you haven't used before. A small window of previous encounters will be displayed. Compare your screen to the window shown in the center of Figure 8-3.

Select "5/11/2012 10:45 AM (Office Visit)." The encounter note from that date will be displayed.

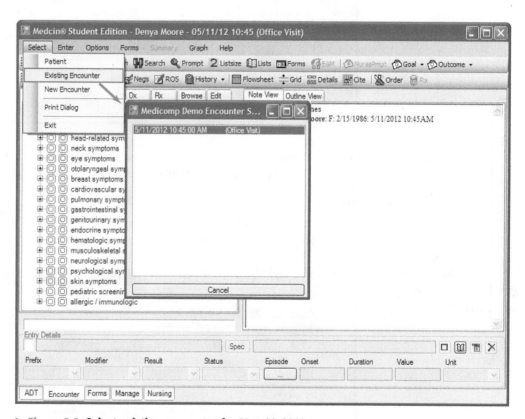

Figure 8-3 Select existing encounter for May 11, 2012.

Step 3

Compare your screen to Figure 8-4. The exam was created using the Adult URI list and therefore should look familiar to you.

Because this is the first time that you have retrieved a previous encounter, and because we are going to be using the information from the encounter note to calculate the E&M code, take a few minutes to look at the encounter note in the right pane of your screen.

Pay attention to the History section. It contains Review of Systems, but no HPI or social history; this will be discussed later in this exercise.

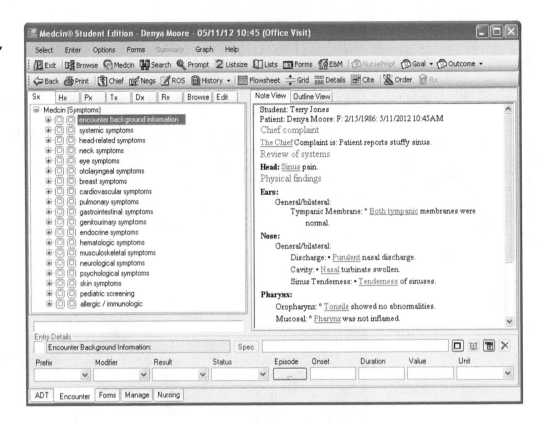

▶ Figure 8-4 **Patient encounter note for May 11, 2012, encounter.**

Not all of the note will fit in the pane, so you will need to use the scroll bar on the right to scroll downward to see the rest of the note, as shown in Figure 8-5.

Step 4

Compare the number of body systems in the Physical Findings section with the number of systems in Review of Systems section.

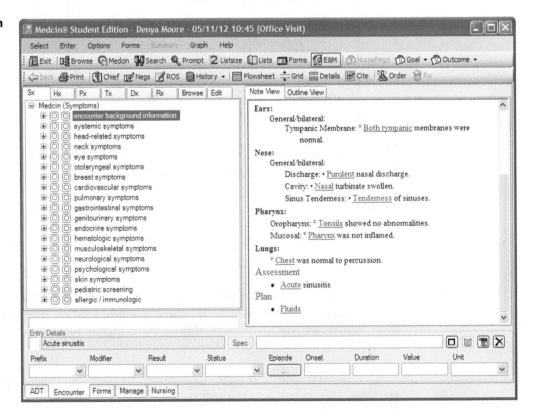

▶ Figure 8-5 **Scrolled portion of patient encounter note for May 11, 2012.**

When you are sufficiently familiar with the encounter note, locate the button labeled "E&M" in the Toolbar at the top of your screen. The icon resembles a horseshoe magnet with a lightning bolt. It is highlighted in the Toolbar on Figure 8-5.

Click on the E&M button to invoke the E&M Calculator window. The first screen that will be displayed is the Problem Screening checklist shown in Figure 8-6.

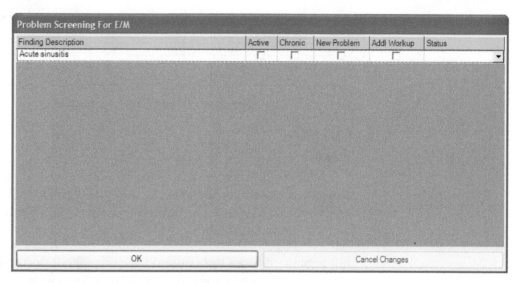

▶ Figure 8-6 **Problem Screening checklist window.**

Problem Screening Checklist Window

Certain E&M calculations are affected by factors of the problem assessment that may not be explicitly documented in the encounter note such as:

◆ Is the problem active or inactive?

◆ Is the problem chronic or not?

◆ Is the problem new to the examiner?

◆ Is additional workup planned for the problem?

◆ Is the problem stable or worsening?

The Problem Screening checklist (shown in Figure 8-6) displays assessments in the current encounter. Providers can add information for the E&M Calculator about each problem by checking boxes for active, chronic, new, or additional workup. A drop-down list lets the provider inform the E&M Calculator of the problem status, but this does not alter a problem status entered via the Entry Detail Status field.

Step 5

We will explore the effect of this window later as we discuss problem risk and management.

Do not check any of the boxes at this time. Locate and click on the OK button on the bottom of the Problem Screening for E/M window. The Evaluation and Management Calculator window will be displayed (as shown in Figure 8-7.)

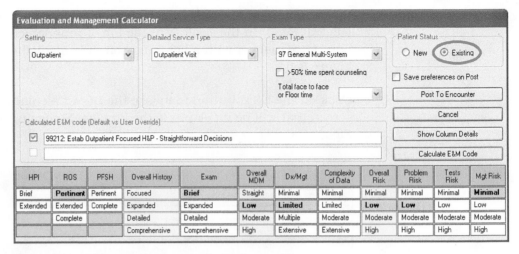

Evaluation and Management Calculator

HPI	ROS	PFSH	Overall History	Exam	Overall MDM	Dx/Mgt	Complexity of Data	Overall Risk	Problem Risk	Tests Risk	Mgt Risk
Brief	**Pertinent**	Pertinent	Focused	**Brief**	Straight	Minimal	Minimal	Minimal	Minimal	Minimal	**Minimal**
Extended	Extended	Complete	Expanded	Expanded	**Low**	**Limited**	Limited	**Low**	**Low**	Low	Low
	Complete		Detailed	Detailed	Moderate	Multiple	Moderate	Moderate	Moderate	Moderate	Moderate
			Comprehensive	Comprehensive	High	Extensive	Extensive	High	High	High	High

▶ Figure 8-7 **E&M Calculator for May 11, 2012, encounter.**

Step 6

The fields in this screen will be explained in Exercise 39; for the moment, we will just calculate the E&M code. If the field labeled "Calculated E&M code" displays "99212 Estab Outpatient Focused H&P—Straightforward Decisions," you are ready to proceed.

If it is blank or does not contain the code 99212, locate the area labeled "Patient Status" in the upper right corner. If the white circle next to "Existing" is empty, click it once with your mouse. The center of the circle should then fill (as shown in Figure 8-7, circled in red). Locate the large button labeled "Calculate E&M Code" and click it. (The button is highlighted in Figure 8-7.)

Compare your screen to the Evaluation and Management Calculator window shown in Figure 8-7.

Step 7

You are going to use the E&M Calculator window to help you understand the CMS's *Documentation Guidelines for Evaluation and Management Services.*

Look at the bottom of the calculator window at the grid. The columns are labeled with terms you may recognize such as HPI and ROS. There are four rows representing the four levels discussed earlier. Each of the columns lists the levels relevant to that particular type of finding. This will be explained further later in this chapter.

Leave your E&M Calculator displayed as you read the following section. Do not click any more buttons until instructed to do so. If you cannot complete the reading in the allotted time, simply repeat steps 1, 2, 4, and 5 to invoke the E&M Calculator window again when you are ready to resume.

Levels of Key Components

You will recall from an earlier discussion that *history, examination,* and *medical decision making* are the key components that determine the level of E&M services.

The CPT-4 E&M code description lists the three key components and their levels. For example:

> 99212 "Established Patient, Focused History and Physical, Straightforward Decision Making."

The key components each have levels of their own, which are determined separately. Components have a numerical level of 1 to 4 and they also have a name, such as *brief, extended, low, high, simple,* or *complex.* The level of E&M code is derived from the highest level of two or three key components.

Key Component: History

The History component includes the following elements:

◆ **CC**, which is an acronym for "chief complaint." A chief complaint is required for all levels of History.

◆ **HPI**, which is an acronym for history of present illness.

◆ **ROS**, which is an acronym for review of systems.

◆ **PFSH**, which is an acronym for past history, family history, and social history.

The extent of history of present illness, review of systems, and past, family, or social history that is obtained and documented is dependent on clinical judgment and the nature of the presenting problems.

Step 8

Look at the grid section of the E&M Calculator window shown in Figure 8-8. The History section consists of columns labeled "HPI," "ROS," "PFSH," and "Overall History."

► Figure 8-8 **History section of E&M Calculator with Show Column Details button highlighted.**

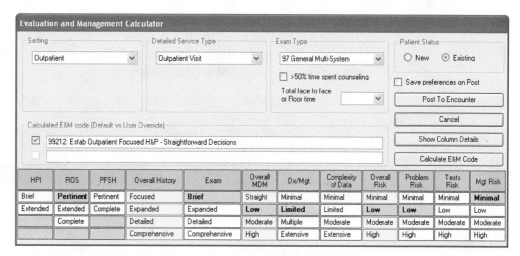

Each of the history elements (HPI, ROS, PFSH) has levels that will determine the Overall History level. If the level in a column is shown in bold type, then the number of findings is sufficient to meet the guidelines for the level at which it appears. For example, look at the column labeled "ROS." The word "**Pertinent**" in the first row is bold, meaning ROS has enough findings for level 1 but not enough for level 2, "Extended."

We now discuss the history elements and levels.

History of Present Illness (HPI) The HPI is a chronological description of the development of the patient's present illness from the first sign and/or symptom or from the previous encounter to the present. HPI includes the following characteristics:

◆ Location

◆ Quality

◆ Severity

◆ Duration

◆ Timing

◆ Context

◆ Modifying factors

◆ Associated signs and symptoms

HPI has two named levels, brief and extended. The levels are determined by the quantity of findings:

Brief: consists of one to three items in the HPI

Extended: consists of at least four items in the HPI or the status of at least three chronic or inactive conditions

In this encounter, there are no findings for HPI; therefore none of the levels are in bold type.

Step 9

The E&M Calculator will allow you to see which findings in the encounter note were used to determine the level. There are two ways to do this.

The first is by using the button labeled "Show Column Details" (highlighted in Figure 8-8). Clicking on that button will display a drop-down list. Selecting the name of a column from this list will display a list of findings from the encounter note that are relevant to that column.

Locate and click on the button labeled "Show Column Details."

Position your mouse over "Details for ROS" in the drop-down list, as shown in Figure 8-9, and click the mouse.

▶ Figure 8-9 **Show Column Details drop-down list.**

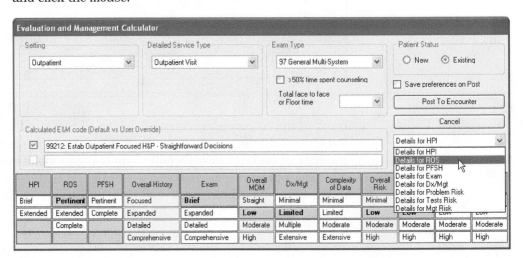

A pane will open in the upper portion of the E&M Calculator window to display the findings that were recorded in the encounter note for Review of Systems (ROS) (as shown in Figure 8-10).

► Figure 8-10 **ROS details in E&M Calculator with Hide Details button highlighted.**

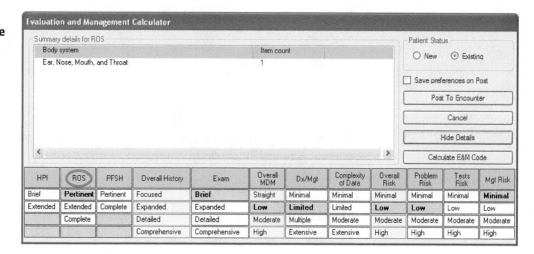

HPI	ROS	PFSH	Overall History	Exam	Overall MDM	Dx/Mgt	Complexity of Data	Overall Risk	Problem Risk	Tests Risk	Mgt Risk
Brief	**Pertinent**	Pertinent	Focused	**Brief**	Straight	Minimal	Minimal	Minimal	Minimal	Minimal	**Minimal**
Extended	Extended	Complete	Expanded	Expanded	**Low**	**Limited**	Limited	**Low**	**Low**	Low	Low
	Complete		Detailed	Detailed	Moderate	Multiple	Moderate	Moderate	Moderate	Moderate	Moderate
			Comprehensive	Comprehensive	High	Extensive	Extensive	High	High	High	High

The second method of displaying column details is to click your mouse directly on the column label, for example, "ROS" (circled in red in Figure 8-10).

Using either method will change the button label to "Hide Details." Clicking the button will close the detail pane and return to the previous view.

Step 10

Review of Systems (ROS) The ROS level is determined by the number of systems reviewed. ROS has three levels:

Problem Pertinent: ROS inquires about the system directly related to the problems identified in the HPI.

Extended: ROS inquires about the system directly related to the problems identified in the HPI and a number of additional systems. Extended level requires two to nine systems be documented.

Complete: ROS inquires about the systems directly related to the problems identified in the HPI plus all additional body systems. At least 10 organ systems must be reviewed to meet the requirement for Complete.

Compare your screen to Figure 8-10. One finding is shown in Figure 8-10; therefore, the ROS is level 1, Pertinent.

Close the Details for ROS pane and return to the previous view by clicking the button labeled "Hide Details" (highlighted in Figure 8-10). Be careful not to click the Cancel button by mistake, because that will close the E&M Calculator instead of hiding the details of ROS.

Step 11

Past, Family, and/or Social History (PFSH) The PFSH consists of a review of three areas:

◆ **Past history:** the patient's past experiences with illnesses, operations, injuries, and treatments

◆ **Family history:** a review of medical events in the patient's family, including diseases that may be hereditary or place the patient at risk

◆ **Social history:** an age-appropriate review of past and current activities

PFSH level is determined by the number of findings in these three history types. PFSH has two levels, level 3 and level 4:

Pertinent: at least one item in any PFSH area directly related to the problems identified in the HPI

Complete: a review of two or all three of the PFSH history areas, depending on the category of the E&M service. Complete requires all three history areas for services that include a comprehensive assessment of a new patient or reassessment of an existing patient. A review of two of the three history areas is sufficient for other services.

In this encounter no PFSH was recorded.

Step 12

The key component History has four levels:

1. Problem Focused

2. Expanded Problem Focused

3. Detailed

4. Comprehensive

Figure 8-11 shows the elements required for each level of history. The level of History is determined by the levels of the HPI, ROS, and PFSH elements.

Compare Figure 8-11 to the HPI, ROS, and PFSH columns on your screen. The fifth column in the E&M Calculator grid, labeled "Overall History," is comparable to the first column in Figure 8-11, Level of History.

▶ **Figure 8-11 Table of Elements Required for Each Level of History.**

Table of Elements Required for Each Level of History

	Level of History	CC	History of Present Illness (HPI)	Review of Systems (ROS)	Past, Family, and/or Social History (PFSH)
			History Elements		
1	Problem Focused	*	Brief (1–3 elements)	(No elements required)	(No elements required)
2	Expanded Problem Focused	*	Brief (1–3 elements)	Problem Pertinent (related to HPI)	(No elements required)
3	Detailed	*	Extended (4 or more)	Extended (2–9 body systems)	Pertinent (1 or more)
4	Comprehensive	*	Extended (4 or more)	Complete (10 or more body systems)	Complete (2 areas Past, Family, or Social)

* Chief Complaint is expected for all Types of History.

Looking at the chart in Figure 8-11, do you see why the overall history is not level 1? It is because only ROS has been recorded, and HPI is required.

Key Component: Examination

The next key component is the Physical Examination. Examination guidelines have been defined for a general multisystem exam and the following 10 single-organ systems:

◆ Cardiovascular

◆ Ears, nose, and throat

◆ Eyes

◆ Genitourinary (female or male)

◆ Hematologic/lymphatic/immunologic

◆ Musculoskeletal

◆ Neurological

◆ Psychiatric

◆ Respiratory

◆ Skin

A general multisystem examination or a single-organ system examination may be performed by any physician, regardless of specialty. The type and content of examination are selected by the examining physician and are based on clinical judgment, the patient's history, and the nature of the presenting problems.

There are four levels of any type of examination:

Brief: a problem-focused, limited examination of the affected body area or organ system

Expanded: a problem-focused, limited examination of the affected body area or organ system and any other symptomatic or related body areas or organ systems

Detailed: an extended examination of the affected body areas or organ systems and any other symptomatic or related body areas or organ systems

Comprehensive: a general multisystem examination, or complete examination of a single organ system and other symptomatic or related body areas or organ systems

The required elements for different levels of single-organ system exams and the general multisystem exam vary; therefore, separate tables are published for each type of system. An abridged example of the Elements of General Multisystem Examination table has been reprinted in Figure 8-12.[4]

Within the guideline tables, individual elements of the examination pertaining to a body area or organ system are identified by bullets. A bullet is a typographic character that looks like this: • (a solid black circle). Locate the bullets in the second column of Figure 8-12.

---

[4] 1997 *Documentation Guidelines for Evaluation and Management Services*, U.S. Department of Health and Human Services, 1997.

Elements of General Multisystem Examination

System/Body Area	Exam Elements
Constitutional	• Measurement of any three of the following seven vital signs: (1) sitting or standing blood pressure, (2) supine blood pressure, (3) pulse rate and regularity, (4) respiration, (5) temperature, (6) height, (7) weight (may be measured and recorded by ancillary staff) • General appearance of patient (e.g., development, nutrition, body habitus, deformities, attention to grooming)
Eyes	• Inspection of conjunctivae and lids • Examination of pupils and irises (e.g., reaction to light and accommodation, size and symmetry) • Ophthalmoscopic examination of optic discs (e.g., size, C/D ratio, appearance) and posterior segments (e.g., vessel changes, exudates, hemorrhages)
Ears, Nose, Mouth, and Throat	• External inspection of ears and nose (e.g., overall appearance, scars, lesions, masses) • Otoscopic examination of external auditory canals and tympanic membranes • Assessment of hearing (e.g., whispered voice, finger rub, tuning fork) • Inspection of nasal mucosa, septum, and turbinates • Inspection of lips, teeth, and gums • Examination of oropharynx: oral mucosa, salivary glands, hard and soft palates, tongue, tonsils, and posterior pharynx
Neck	• Examination of neck (e.g., masses, overall appearance, symmetry, tracheal position, crepitus) • Examination of thyroid (e.g., enlargement, tenderness, mass)
Respiratory	• Assessment of respiratory effort (e.g., intercostal retractions, use of accessory muscles, diaphragmatic movement) • Percussion of chest (e.g., dullness, flatness, hyperresonance) • Palpation of chest (e.g., tactile fremitus) • Auscultation of lungs (e.g., breath sounds, adventitious sounds, rubs)
Cardiovascular	• Palpation of heart (e.g., location, size, thrills) • Auscultation of heart with notation of abnormal sounds and murmurs Examination of: • carotid arteries (e.g., pulse amplitude, bruits) • abdominal aorta (e.g., size, bruits) • femoral arteries (e.g., pulse amplitude, bruits) • pedal pulses (e.g., pulse amplitude) • extremities for edema and/or varicosities
Chest (Breasts)	• Inspection of breasts (e.g., symmetry, nipple discharge) • Palpation of breasts and axillae (e.g., masses or lumps, tenderness)
Gastrointestinal (Abdomen)	• Examination of abdomen with notation of presence of masses or tenderness • Examination of liver and spleen • Examination for presence or absence of hernia • Examination (when indicated) of anus, perineum and rectum, including sphincter tone, presence of hemorrhoids, rectal masses • Obtain stool sample for occult blood test when indicated

If you have taken a class in medical coding or read the CPT-4 book you may be familiar with the concept of "the number of bullets required to meet a level of E&M coding." This simply means how many findings in the encounter note correspond to elements in the guideline table with bullet characters printed next to them.

Step 13

Locate and click on the column labeled "Exam" (as shown in Figure 8-13). The grid has only one column for the Exam component. A pane displaying the exam details will open in the E&M Calculator window.

▶ Figure 8-13 **Exam details of E&M Calculator.**

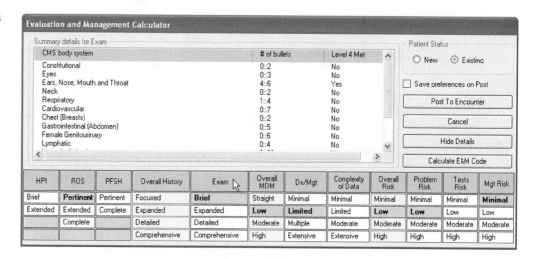

The Summary Details for Exam pane has three columns, labeled "CMS body system," "# of bullets," and "Level 4 Met." (The "bullets" referred to are quite literally the typographic characters printed in the table in Figure 8-12.)

Each row under the column labeled "# of bullets" has a pair of numbers. For example, locate the row for Ears, Nose, Mouth and Throat; you will see the numbers 4:6. This means the clinician examined four of six elements in that system.

Step 14

Compare your screen with the table in Figure 8-14. You will see five elements with bullets documented in the exam (four bullets in Ear, Nose, Mouth and Throat and 1 bullet in Respiratory). Therefore the examination is level 1, "Problem Focused Exam," because there are only five bullets.

The Exam level is not determined by the number of findings but by the number of bullets satisfied within a system/body area. Findings do not have to be abnormal; normal findings count as well.

Key Component: Medical Decision Making

The third key component is medical decision making. The remaining columns in the E&M Calculator window grid are all concerned with medical decision making. Medical decision making (MDM) refers to the complexity of establishing a diagnosis or selecting a management option as measured by three elements:

◆ **Number of possible diagnoses or management options** This element has four levels. The level is determined by the number and types of problems

Table of Elements Required for Each Level of Examination

	Level of Examination	Examination Elements by Type of Exam	
		General Multisystem Examinations	Single Organ System Examinations
1	*Problem Focused* (Brief)	1 to 5 elements identified by a bullet (•) in one or more organ systems or body areas.	1 to 5 elements identified by a bullet (•), whether in a box with a shaded or unshaded border.*
2	*Expanded Problem Focused*	At least 6 elements identified by a bullet (•) in one or more organ systems or body areas.	At least 6 elements identified by a bullet (•), whether in a box with a shaded or unshaded border.*
3	*Detailed Examination*	At least 6 organ systems or body areas; for each system/area selected at least 2 elements identified by a bullet (•). Alternatively, at least 12 elements identified by a bullet (•) in 2 or more organ systems or body areas.	At least 12 elements identified by a bullet (•), whether in a box with a shaded or unshaded border.* Exception: requirement reduced to 9 elements for Eye and psychiatric examinations.
4	*Comprehensive Examination*	At least 9 organ systems or body areas; for each system/area selected all elements identified by a bullet (•).	Every element in each box with a shaded border and at least 1 element in each box with an unshaded border; Plus all elements identified by a bullet (•) whether in a box with a shaded or unshaded border.*

* This refers to sections of the printed tables for Single Organ System Exams, which are outlined with a shaded border.

addressed during the encounter, the complexity of establishing a diagnosis, and the management decisions that are made by the physician. The levels include:

Level 1: **Minimal**

Level 2: **Limited**

Level 3: **Multiple**

Level 4: **Extensive**

◆ **Amount or Complexity of Data to Be Reviewed** There are four levels for this element as well, including:

Level 1: **Minimal** or None

Level 2: **Limited**

Level 3: **Moderate**

Level 4: **Extensive**

◆ **Risk of Significant Complications, Morbidity, or Mortality** This element is based on the risks associated with the presenting problems, the diagnostic procedures, and the possible management options. Risk also has four levels:

Level 1: **Minimal**

Level 2: **Low**

Level 3: **Moderate**

Level 4: **High**

As you can see, each of the elements of medical decision making has four levels. The overall level of the MDM component is derived from the highest level of two of the three elements. This is shown in the column labeled "Overall MDM" in the E&M Calculator window. Let us look at how it was determined.

Step 15

Locate and click on the column labeled "Dx/Mgt" (as shown in Figure 8-15). "Dx/Mgt" stands for Diagnosis and/or Management options. The E&M Calculator window will display the "Details for Dx/Mgt" pane.

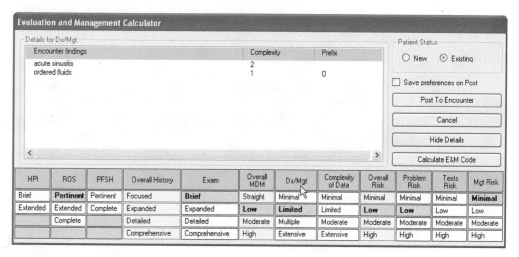

▶ Figure 8-15 **Medical decision making—details for Dx/Mgt.**

The details pane has three columns, labeled "Encounter findings," "Complexity," and "Prefix." The Complexity column displays a level of complexity associated with the finding. The Prefix column contains a code or abbreviation if the finding has a prefix. In this example, the finding "ordered fluids" displays the letter "O," which stands for ordered.

Step 16

The remaining columns in the E&M Calculator window grid are concerned with the MDM element of risk.

Locate and click on the column labeled "Problem Risk" as shown in Figure 8-16. The E&M Calculator window will display the "Details for Problem Risk" pane.

The details pane has three columns, labeled "Encounter findings," "Risk level," and "Prefix," which were explained in the previous step.

Step 17

Locate and click on the column labeled "Mgt Risk" (as shown in Figure 8-17). "Mgt" is the software abbreviation for "management." The pane in the E&M Calculator window will display the Details for Mgt Risk pane.

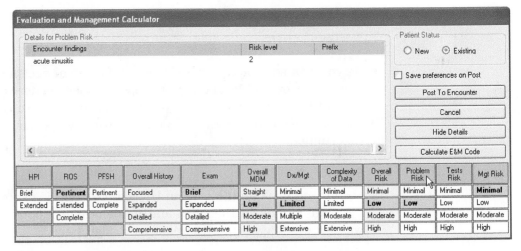

▶ Figure 8-16 **Medical decision making—details for Problem Risk.**

Details for Problem Risk

Encounter findings	Risk level	Prefix
acute sinusitis	2	

Patient Status: ○ New ◉ Existing

☐ Save preferences on Post

Post To Encounter

Cancel

Hide Details

Calculate E&M Code

HPI	ROS	PFSH	Overall History	Exam	Overall MDM	Dx/Mgt	Complexity of Data	Overall Risk	Problem Risk	Tests Risk	Mgt Risk
Brief	**Pertinent**	Pertinent	Focused	**Brief**	Straight	Minimal	Minimal	Minimal	Minimal	Minimal	**Minimal**
Extended	Extended	Complete	Expanded	Expanded	**Low**	**Limited**	Limited	**Low**	**Low**	Low	Low
	Complete		Detailed	Detailed	Moderate	Multiple	Moderate	Moderate	Moderate	Moderate	Moderate
			Comprehensive	Comprehensive	High	Extensive	Extensive	High	High	High	High

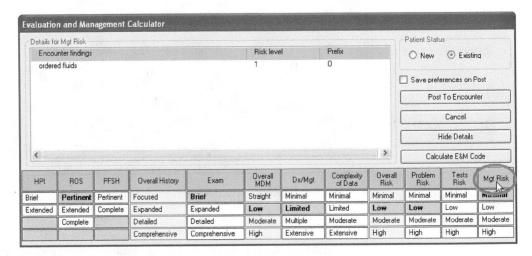

▶ Figure 8-17 **Medical decision making—details for Mgt Risk.**

Details for Mgt Risk

Encounter findings	Risk level	Prefix
ordered fluids	1	0

Patient Status: ○ New ◉ Existing

☐ Save preferences on Post

Post To Encounter

Cancel

Hide Details

Calculate E&M Code

HPI	ROS	PFSH	Overall History	Exam	Overall MDM	Dx/Mgt	Complexity of Data	Overall Risk	Problem Risk	Tests Risk	Mgt Risk
Brief	**Pertinent**	Pertinent	Focused	**Brief**	Straight	Minimal	Minimal	Minimal	Minimal	Minimal	Minimal
Extended	Extended	Complete	Expanded	Expanded	**Low**	**Limited**	Limited	**Low**	**Low**	Low	Low
	Complete		Detailed	Detailed	Moderate	Multiple	Moderate	Moderate	Moderate	Moderate	Moderate
			Comprehensive	Comprehensive	High	Extensive	Extensive	High	High	High	High

The details pane has three columns, labeled "Encounter findings," "Risk Level," and "Prefix," which were explained in step 15. In this example there is "Minimal" risk when ordering fluids. The E&M Calculator also includes a column measuring the risk of tests, but none were ordered during this encounter.

Step 18

The E&M guidelines use a special table for calculating the overall level of risk (shown in Figure 8-18). However, risk differs from the other two MDM elements in that risk level is the highest level of any *one* column in the table.

The table in Figure 8-18 is used to determine whether the risk of significant complications, morbidity, or mortality is minimal, low, moderate, or high. Because the determination of risk is complex and not readily quantifiable, the table includes common clinical examples rather than absolute measures of risk.

Table of Risk

Level of Risk	Presenting Problem(s)	Diagnostic Procedure(s) Ordered	Management Options Selected
1 Minimal	• One self-limited or minor problem, e.g., cold, insect bite, tinea corporis	• Laboratory tests requiring venipuncture • Chest x-rays • EKG/EEG • Urinalysis • Ultrasound, e.g., echocardiography • KOH prep	• Rest • Gargles • Elastic bandages • Superficial dressings
2 Low	• Two or more self-limited or minor problems • One stable chronic illness, e.g., well-controlled hypertension, non–insulin dependent diabetes, cataract, BPH • Acute uncomplicated illness or injury, e.g., cystitis, allergic rhinitis, simple sprain	• Physiologic tests not under stress, e.g., pulmonary function tests • Non-cardiovascular imaging studies with contrast, e.g., barium enema • Superficial needle biopsies • Clinical laboratory tests requiring arterial puncture • Skin biopsies	• Over-the-counter drugs • Minor surgery with no identified risk factors • Physical therapy • Occupational therapy • IV fluids without additives
3 Moderate	• One or more chronic illnesses with mild exacerbation, progression, or side effects of treatment • Two or more stable chronic illnesses • Undiagnosed new problem with uncertain prognosis, e.g., lump in breast • Acute illness with systemic symptoms, e.g., pyelonephritis, pneumonitis, colitis • Acute complicated injury, e.g., head injury with brief loss of consciousness	• Physiologic tests under stress, e.g., cardiac stress test, fetal contraction stress test • Diagnostic endoscopies with no identified risk factors • Deep needle or incisional biopsy • Cardiovascular imaging studies with contrast and no identified risk factors, e.g., arteriogram, cardiac catheterization • Obtain fluid from body cavity, e.g., lumbar puncture, thoracentesis, culdocentesis	• Minor surgery with identified risk factors • Elective major surgery (open, percutaneous, or endoscopic) with no identified risk factors • Prescription drug management • Therapeutic nuclear medicine • IV fluids with additives • Closed treatment of fracture or dislocation without manipulation
4 High	• One or more chronic illnesses with severe exacerbation, progression, or side effects of treatment • Acute or chronic illnesses or injuries that pose a threat to life or bodily function, e.g., multiple trauma, acute MI, pulmonary embolus, severe respiratory distress, progressive severe rheumatoid arthritis, psychiatric illness with potential threat to self or others, peritonitis, acute renal failure • An abrupt change in neurologic status, e.g., seizure, TIA, weakness, sensory loss	• Cardiovascular imaging studies with contrast with identified risk factors • Cardiac electrophysiological tests • Diagnostic endoscopies with identified risk factors • Discography	• Elective major surgery (open, percutaneous, or endoscopic) with identified risk factors • Emergency major surgery (open, percutaneous, or endoscopic) • Parenteral controlled substances • Drug therapy requiring intensive monitoring for toxicity • Decision not to resuscitate or to deescalate care because of poor prognosis

► Figure 8-18 **Table for determining level of risk.**

Locate the column in the E&M Calculator window labeled "Overall Risk." Notice that the level of the Overall Risk column is "low," because that was the level of the highest of the three risk elements, Problem Risk. You will see another example of this aspect of risk in Exercise 39.

Determining the Level of Medical Decision Making

There are four levels of medical decision making:

>   Level 1: **Straight**forward
>
>   Level 2: **Low** Complexity
>
>   Level 3: **Moderate** Complexity
>
>   Level 4: **High** Complexity

The individual levels from each of the elements we have discussed, number of diagnoses, amount or complexity of data, and the level of risk are used to determine the level for MDM.

The chart in Figure 8-19 shows the level of elements required for each level of medical decision making. The level of MDM (shown in the first column) is determined by the highest levels of any *two* of the three elements.

▶ Figure 8-19 **Elements required for each level of medical decision making.**

Table of Levels of Medical Decision Making

Level of MDM	Medical Decision Making	Number of diagnoses or management options	Amount and/or complexity of data to be reviewed	Risk of complications and/or morbidity or mortality
1	*Straightforward*	Minimal	Minimal or None	Minimal
2	*Low Complexity*	Limited	Limited	Low
3	*Moderate Complexity*	Multiple	Moderate	Moderate
4	*High Complexity*	Extensive	Extensive	High

Step 19

Compare the chart in Figure 8-19 to the E&M Calculator window.

Locate the column labeled "Overall MDM", which is "low" or level 2.

Looking at the columns for the individual elements, note that those labeled "Dx/Mgt Options" and "Overall Risk" are also level 2. Even though there is no report for "Complexity of Data," the MDM level is set to the highest of two out of three elements.

Other Components: Counseling, Coordination of Care, and Time

In the case in which counseling or coordination of care dominates (more than 50%) the physician/patient or family encounter (face-to-face time in the office or other or outpatient setting, floor/unit time in the hospital or nursing facility), time is considered the key or controlling factor to qualify for a particular level of E&M services.

Step 20

Click on the button labeled "Hide Details" to return to the E&M Calculator screen. (If you have difficulty locating the button, refer to Figure 8-10.)

In the center of the E&M Calculator window, beneath the Exam Type field, are two fields related to time. First is a check box used to indicate that counseling (or coordination of care) exceeded 50% of the face-to-face time for the visit. The second field is a drop-down list used to enter the total face-to-face time.

Face-to-face time incorporates the total time both before and after the visit such as taking patient history, performing the exam, reviewing lab results, planning for follow-up care, and communicating with other providers about the patient's case.

The E&M Calculator allows you to record the amount of face-to-face time even when you are not using counseling time as a factor. It is a good practice to record the face-to-face time for each encounter.

Click on the down arrow button in the field labeled "Total face to face or Floor time" and select 15 minutes from the drop-down list as shown in Figure 8-20.

▶ Figure 8-20 **Counseling and face-to-face time drop-down list.**

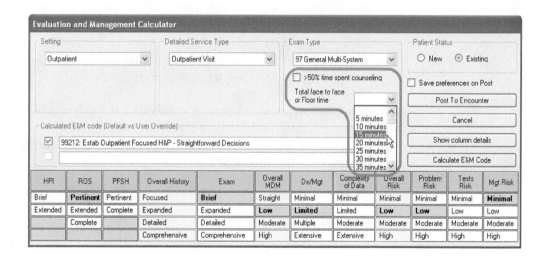

This will not change the E&M code because time does not become a factor until it is more than half of the face-to-face time.

In the next exercise, you will learn to use both of these time-related fields to change the E&M code and to document the results in your encounter note.

Putting It All Together

Momentarily leaving the element of time aside, you will see that the levels of each of the three *key components* combine to determine the level of the E&M code.

The chart in Figure 8-21 shows the CPT-4 E&M codes used for the category of outpatient office visits. It will help you to visualize how the relationship of the key components determines the E&M code.

Relationship of Key Elements to E&M Codes for Outpatient Visits

E&M Code	Type of Patient	# of Key Elements Met	History Level	Exam Level	Medical Decision Making	Face-to-face Time
99201	New	All 3	1	1	1	10 min
99202	New	All 3	2	2	1	20 min
99203	New	All 3	3	3	2	30 min
99204	New	All 3	4	4	3	45 min
99205	New	All 3	4	4	4	60 min
99211	Established	2 of 3	Presentation of Problem Minimal Documentation Req.			5 min
99212	Established	2 of 3	1	1	1	10 min
99213	Established	2 of 3	2	2	2	15 min
99214	Established	2 of 3	3	3	3	25 min
99215	Established	2 of 3	4	4	4	40 min

▶ Figure 8-21 **Relationship of key component levels determines E&M code.**

The first column in Figure 8-21 is the CPT-4 code. The second column indicates whether the code is for use with a new or established patient. Note that two groups of codes are listed. The first five codes are for new patients, and then five different codes are listed for established patients.

The third column labeled "# of Key Elements Met" indicates how many key components determine the E&M code.

The blue, green, and lavender columns list the levels of the three key components: History, Exam, and Medical Decision Making. The level numbers under each key component are derived from the individual tables in the sections you have just completed. The tables are

History—Figure 8-11

Exam—Figure 8-14

MDM—Figure 8-19

The final column lists the number of minutes per type of visit used by the E&M Calculator. Time will be discussed in a subsequent exercise.

Evaluating Key Components

Once the level of each of the key components has been determined, calculating the level of the E&M code is fairly straightforward. The E&M code level is determined by the lowest level of the key components considered. However, different requirements apply when determining the E&M code for new versus established patients.

Scan down the third column of Figure 8-21. Note that the number of key components for new patients is "All 3." Notice that for established patients it is "2 of 3." This doesn't mean that an encounter won't have findings for all three components, but in most cases it will. It means that, for an established patient, the two key components with the highest levels are considered and the lowest level of the two determines the E&M code.

For example, consider an encounter that has:

History Level 1 (Problem Focused)

Exam Level 2 (Expanded Problem Focused)

MDM Level 3 (Moderate Complexity)

The E&M code for an established patient will be level 2 because only Exam and MDM are considered and Exam has the lower level.

If the encounter was for a new patient the E&M code would be level 1 because all three key components are considered and the lowest is History (level 1).

Look at the section of the table for new patients. What E&M code would be used when History is level 1 (Problem Focused), Exam is level 2 (Expanded Problem Focused), and MDM is level 2 (Low Complexity)?

If you answered 99201, you are correct. The E&M code for new patients is determined by all three elements. Even though the Exam and MDM components are level 2, if the History level is not 2, then the lower code must be used.

Having tried to determine the code manually, you can appreciate the value that an E&M Calculator brings to an EHR system. Remember that the level of each of the key components is a combination of elements:

◆ To qualify for a given level of history, the quantity and types of HPI, ROS, and PFSH must be met.

◆ To qualify for a given level of exam, the number of "bulleted" items in the appropriate number of body systems must be met.

◆ To qualify for a given level of medical decision making, two of the three elements (the number of diagnosis, the amount of data, and the risk assessment) must be either met or exceeded.

If you can imagine trying to count bullets from your encounter notes, calculate the amount of and types of history, and determine the level of decision making in your head, all while you are seeing the patient, you can understand why so many doctors code at the wrong level, just to be safe. You also can appreciate the skill required of medical coders who do this manually.

Step 21

Click the Cancel button to close the E&M Calculator window. You may exit the Student Edition software **without printing** an encounter this time because you have not made any changes to the note.

Factors That Affect the E&M Code

At this point, you should have a good understanding on how an E&M code is determined from the key elements of the encounter. However, what changes the exam to the next level is not always apparent.

The level of E&M code for an established patient is dependent on two of three of the *key components*. Merely adding more findings to any one component may bring that component to a higher level, but that does not necessarily mean that the visit as a whole will qualify for the higher level E&M code.

For example, in Exercise 38 an established patient had:

History Level 1 *(Problem Focused)*

Exam Level 1 *(Problem Focused)*

MDM Level 2 *(Low Complexity)*

The E&M code was level 1 (99212) because one of the two highest key components was a level 1. Even if the level of MDM was raised to three, the E&M code would still be level 1 because the exam component was only level 1.

Work must be performed and documented in the appropriate areas to result in a higher E&M code. The next exercise demonstrates how changes to key components affect an increase to the level of an E&M code.

In the next exercise, you are going to add findings to an existing encounter to study the effects on E&M coding.

Fraud and Abuse

The goal of these exercises is to provide an experiential understanding of concepts discussed in this chapter. They should not be construed as having any other purpose.

It is unethical and illegal to maximize payment by means that contradict regulatory guidelines. The HHS Office of Inspector General (OIG) investigates allegations of medical billing fraud and abuse. It does not matter if coding errors are made deliberately or inadvertently; OIG still treats it as fraud and abuse.

The student should not get the impression that it is okay to upcode to maximize reimbursement unless legally entitled by documentation and service provided. Similarly, a clinician cannot adjust the time factor unless it is substantiated in the documentation. Diagnoses or procedures should not be inappropriately included or excluded to affect or alter payment or insurance policy coverage requirements.

EHR systems support accurate, complete, and consistent coding practices by documenting the encounter with codified nomenclature that can be analyzed and used to determine the levels of billing justified. Medical coders must adhere to the coding conventions, official coding guidelines, and official rules, and assign codes that are clearly and consistently supported by clinical documentation in the health record.

Guided Exercise 39: Calculating E&M for a More Complex Visit

Step 1

If the patient encounter used in the previous exercise is not currently displayed on your screen, start the Student Edition software.

From the Select Menu, click Patient, and from the Patient Selector window select Denya Moore. If you have difficulty, refer to Figure 8-2 at the beginning of this chapter.

From the Select Menu, click "Existing Encounter," and from the Encounter Selector window select "5/11/2012 10:45 AM (Office Visit)." If you have difficulty, refer to Figure 8-3 at the beginning of this chapter.

You will recall from Exercise 38 that this patient encounter note produces a calculated E&M code of "99212 Established Outpatient Focused H&P—Straightforward Decisions." You do not need to run the E&M Calculator yet.

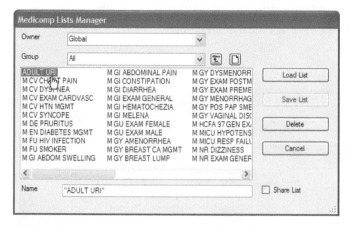

▶ Figure 8-22 **Select the Adult URI list from the Lists Manager window.**

Step 2

The encounter note that you have selected was for an Adult URI and was created using the List feature, which you learned in Chapter 6.

From the Toolbar at the top your screen, click on the button labeled "List."

When the Lists Manager window shown in Figure 8-22 is displayed, select "Adult URI" and click the button labeled "Load List."

In the following steps, you are going to use the list to add findings and study their effect on the levels of E&M codes.

History   The History level is determined by the relationship between HPI, ROS, and PFSH. If you refer back to Figure 8-11, you will see the following:

◆ An increase in the number of findings for HPI will only affect the level of history if ROS and PFSH contain data as well.

◆ An increase in the number of body systems in ROS will only affect the level of history if HPI contains at least four findings and PFSH contains at least one.

◆ Adding even one finding for PFSH will only affect the level of history if HPI contains at least four findings and ROS contains at least two body systems.

◆ A "Complete" level of PFSH will only affect the overall history level when HPI contains at least four findings and ROS has at least 10 systems.

▶ Figure 8-23 **Upper portion of encounter note with Review of Systems section circled in red.**

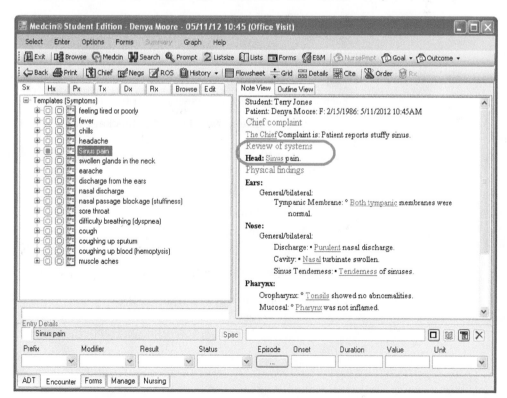

Step 3

Scroll the encounter note, displayed in the pane on the right, upward to view the History section (circled in red in Figure 8-23). Note that there are no HPI or PFSH findings in the History section. This means that there is only one of the three History elements in the current calculation.

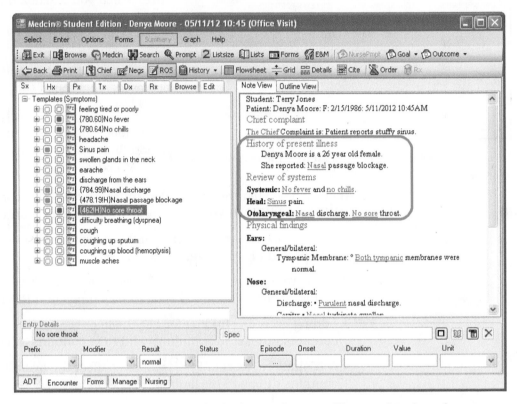

▶ Figure 8-24 **Encounter note with both History of present illness and Review of systems sections.**

Step 4

Locate and click on the following symptom findings:

- (red button) Nasal passage blockage (stuffiness)

Locate the button labeled "ROS" on the Toolbar at the top of the screen and click it.

Locate and click on the following symptom findings:

- (blue button) Fever
- (blue button) Chills
- (red button) Nasal Discharge
- (blue button) Sore Throat

Compare your screen to Figure 8-24.

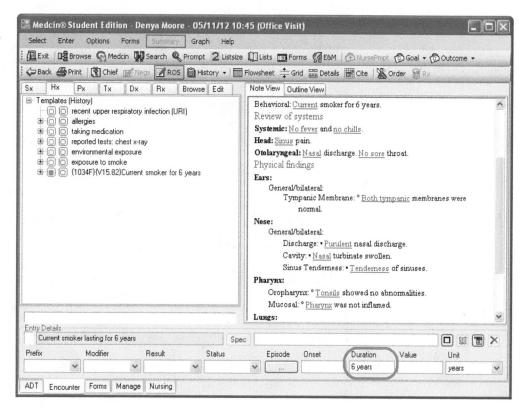

Step 5

Click on the Hx tab.

Locate and click on the following History finding:

● (red button) current smoker

In the Entry Details section at the bottom of your screen, type **6 years** in the field labeled "Duration" (circled in red in Figure 8-25).

Compare your screen to Figure 8-25. Note that you now have findings in all three History sections: HPI, ROS, and behavioral history (PFSH).

Examination Exams provide the most direct but not the easiest means to reach a higher level code. The more systems you examine, or in "single-organ" exams the more bullet points you meet in a single area, the more work you are doing and therefore the higher level of code you should be able to bill for.

◆ In a general multisystem examination, six or more elements with a bullet are required to reach the second level.

◆ The third level is reached when you have at least two elements in six or more systems/body areas.

◆ The fourth level requires all of the bulleted items in at least nine systems/body areas.

Step 6

Click on the Px tab.

Locate and click on the following Physical Exam findings:

● (blue button) Wheezing
● (blue button) Rhonchi

Compare your screen to Figure 8-26.

▶ Figure 8-26 **Added findings on physical exam.**

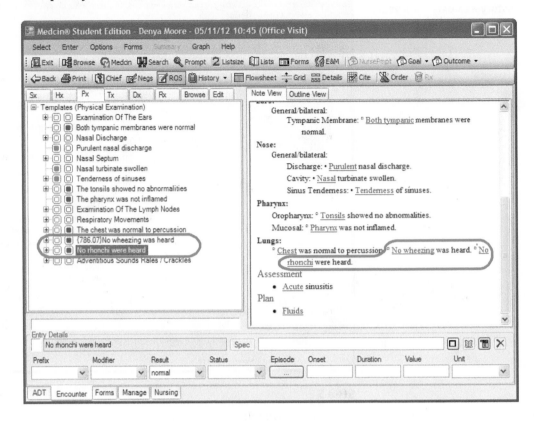

Step 7

Enter the patient's vital signs using the Vitals form. Ms. Moore's vital signs are as follows:

Temperature:	**98**
Respiration:	**15**
Pulse:	**68**
BP:	**128/90**
Height:	**65**
Weight:	**155**

When you have entered all of the vital signs, compare your screen to Figure 8-27 and then click your mouse on the Encounter tab at the bottom of the screen.

Step 8

Click on the E&M button in the Toolbar at the top of your screen. When the Problem Screening checklist window appears, click the OK button without checking any of the boxes. The Evaluation and Management Calculator window should now display the code 99213. If it does not, locate the section labeled Patient Status in the upper right corner of the calculator window. Click on the circle next to the label "Existing" and then click on the button labeled "Calculate E&M Code."

Figure 8-28 shows the E&M code generated as a result of the additional findings you have added. The new code is "99213: Estab Outpatient Expanded H&P—Low Complexity Decisions." Figure 8-20 shows the previously calculated E&M code of 99212. Compare the grid at the bottom of your E&M Calculator window to Figure 8-20.

► Figure 8-27 **Vital signs for Denya Moore.**

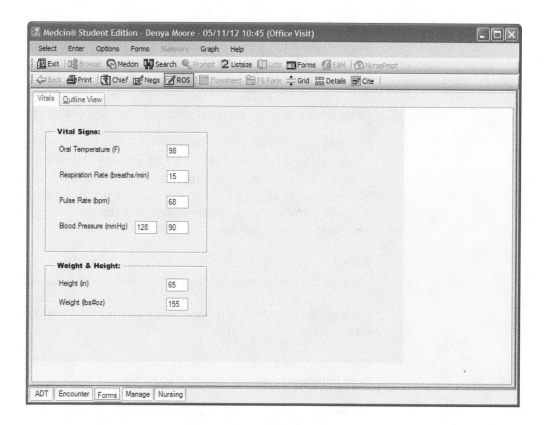

► Figure 8-28 **Recalculated E&M code.**

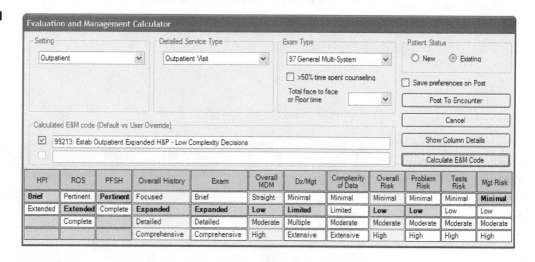

Note that the History sections HPI and PFSH now have bold levels listed in them. Although only the ROS history element moved to level 2, the Overall History level changed from 1–Problem Focused to 2–Expanded Problem Focused. This is because of the presence of the HPI finding and the six ROS findings related to the problem. The addition of the PFSH did not, however, affect the Overall History level. Refer to Figure 8-11, Table of Elements Required for Each Level of History.

Now, notice that the level of Exam has also increased to level 2, Expanded. This was a result of the addition of vital signs and two Physical Exam findings.

Why, if none of the key components changed to level 3, did the E&M code change from a level 2 code (99212) to a level 3 code (99213)?

Refer back to the chart in Figure 8-21; you will notice that for an established patient, the CPT-4 requirement for 99213 is that two of the three key components are at least level 2. Because Overall History and Exam are now level 2 (Expanded), the encounter justifies a higher level E&M code.

In this exercise, the medical decision-making components did not change levels.

Medical Decision Making The level of MDM is determined by two out of three elements in the table shown in Figure 8-19. However, the risk table in Figure 8-18 indicates that managing prescribed medications raises the risk to level 3. Therefore, the MDM level for any patient on medications will usually be determined by the number of diagnoses and the amount or complexity of data reviewed during the visit.

Step 9

Click on the button labeled "Cancel" to close the E&M Calculator window.

Click on the E&M button in the Toolbar at the top of your screen to restart the E&M Calculator.

This time you are going to enter data in the Problem Screening checklist window before proceeding to the E&M Calculator.

When you click your mouse on the check boxes in the Problem Screening for E/M window, a check mark appears.

Locate and click the boxes for the following:

✓ Active

✓ New Problem

Compare your screen to Figure 8-29.

▶ Figure 8-29 **Problem Screening window with Active and New Problem checked.**

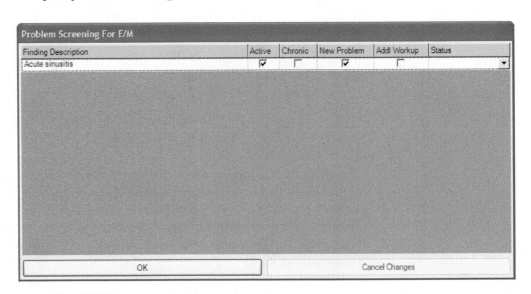

Click the OK button at the bottom of the checklist window.

Step 10

Locate the column labeled "Dx/Mgt." You will recall that Dx/Mgt stands for Diagnosis and/or Management. Compare Figure 8-28 and Figure 8-30.

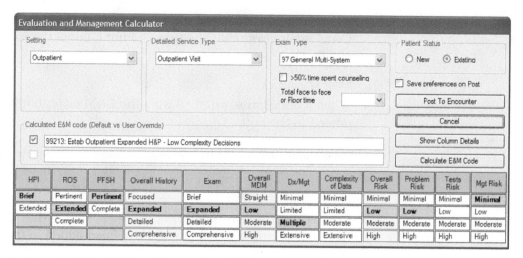

▶ Figure 8-30 **Dx/Mgt level changed to Multiple.**

Notice that the Dx/Mgt column has changed from level 2, Limited, to level 3, Multiple. This change in level was caused by the addition of data from the Problem Screening checklist window.

Time As you learned earlier, time can be a factor when more than 50% of the face-to-face time is spent counseling the patient. Both the face-to-face time and the counseling time must be documented. This is covered later in Exercise 41.

Step 11

Remember that it is always a good idea to record the face-to-face time in the encounter note. The software allows you to do this when you record the E&M code even if you are not using counseling time as a factor in E&M calculation. Remember face-to-face time is the total time you spent on the visit before, during, and after the patient exam. It is not the time spent counseling the patient.

Click on the button with the down arrow in the field labeled "Total face to face or Floor time" and select "15 minutes" (as shown in Figure 8-31).

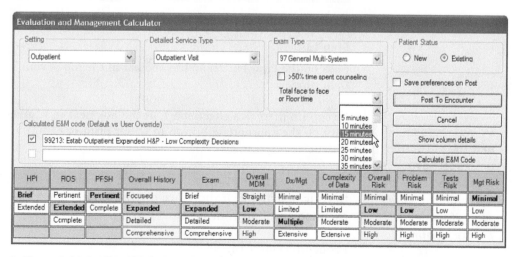

▶ Figure 8-31 **Setting the face-to-face time.**

Recalculate the E&M code by clicking on the button labeled "Calculate E&M Code" again. Note that the time did not change the calculated code, which is still 99213.

Step 12

When a clinician is satisfied with the E&M code that has been calculated, it is posted to the note.

Locate and click on the button labeled "Post To Encounter" (highlighted in Figure 8-31). The E&M Calculator window will close and the E&M code will be added to your note.

Compare your screen with Figure 8-32. Notice that the procedure and the face-to-face time (circled in red) have been added to the bottom of the encounter note.

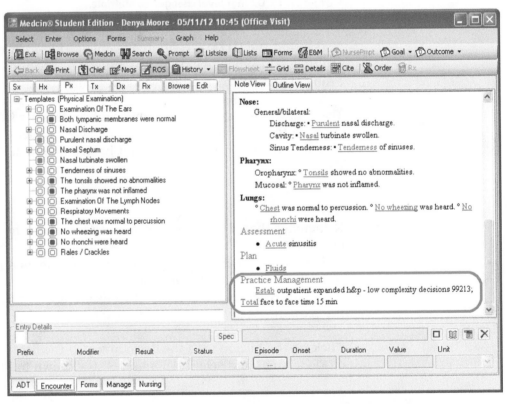

▶ Figure 8-32 **Encounter note with E&M code and face-to-face time circled in red.**

Step 13

Click on the Print button on the Toolbar at the top of your screen to invoke the Print Data window.

Be certain there is a check mark in the box next to "Current Encounter" and then click on the appropriate button to either print or export a file, as directed by your instructor.

Compare your printout or file output to Figure 8-33. If it is correct, hand it in to your instructor. If there are any differences, review the previous steps in the exercise and find your error.

Proceed to step 14.

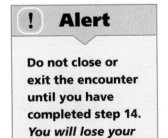

! Alert

Do not close or exit the encounter until you have completed step 14. *You will lose your work if you exit before printing.*

Student: *your name or ID here*
Patient: Denya Moore: F: 2/15/1986: 5/11/2012 10:45 AM
Chief complaint
The Chief Complaint is: Patient reports stuffy sinus.
History of present illness
>   Denya Moore is a 26 year old female.
>   She reported: Nasal passage blockage.
>   Personal history
>   Behavioral: Current smoker for 6 years.

Review of systems
Systemic: No fever and no chills.
Head: Sinus pain.
Otolaryngeal: Nasal discharge. No sore throat.
Physical findings
Vital Signs:

Vital Signs/Measurements	Value	Normal Range
Oral temperature	98 F	97.6 - 99.6
RR	15 breaths/min	18 - 26
PR	68 bpm	50 - 100
Blood pressure	128/90 mmHg	100-120/56-80
Weight	155 lbs	98 - 183
Height	65 in	60.24 - 68.5

Ears:
>   General/bilateral:
>   Tympanic Membrane: ° Both tympanic membranes were normal.

Nose:
>   General/bilateral:
>   Discharge: • Purulent nasal discharge.
>   Cavity: • Nasal turbinate swollen.
>   Sinus Tenderness: • Tenderness of sinuses.

Pharynx:
>   Oropharynx: ° Tonsils showed no abnormalities.
>   Mucosal: ° Pharynx was not inflamed.

Lungs:
>   ° Chest was normal to percussion. ° No wheezing was heard. ° No rhonchi were heard.

Assessment
>   • Acute sinusitis

Plan
>   • Fluids

Practice Management
>   Estab outpatient expanded h&p - low complexity decisions 99213; Total face to face time 15 min

▶ **Figure 8-33 Printed encounter note for Denya Moore, May 11, 2012, 10:45 AM.**

Critical Thinking Exercise 40: Understanding How Procedures Are Posted to the Billing System

EHR systems that are integrated with practice management or billing software can transfer the procedure and diagnosis (CPT-4, HCPCS, and ICD-9-CM) codes from the EHR directly into the practice management billing system.

In most healthcare facilities the codes that are transferred from the EHR do not post automatically to the billing system. Most systems hold these as "pending" charges until they are reviewed by a billing or coding expert who may make modifications to the codes before posting them as charges. Here are few examples of why this is necessary:

◆ Certain procedures are considered part of another procedure (bundled).

◆ Under certain conditions a coding specialist may need to add modifier codes.

◆ Certain codes may represent a supply or sample for which the doctor does not wish to charge the patient.

Step 14

Locate and click on the tab labeled "Outline View" on the right pane of the window. Locate and click the small plus signs next to the folders "Assessment" and "Practice Management."

Compare your screen with Figure 8-34. Notice that the assessment "Acute sinusitis" displays an ICD-9-CM code in this view. Notice also that the text beneath the Practice Management folder not only displays the description information of the calculated E&M code, but the CPT-4 code as well.

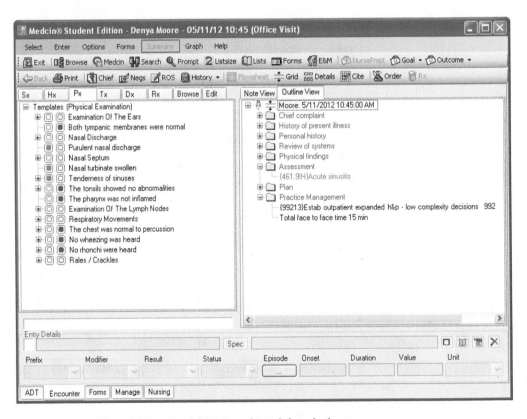

▶ Figure 8-34 Outline View tab with E&M code and description.

Your version of the Student Edition is not connected to a billing system and therefore does not transfer the codes for you. However, it does post codes to the patient encounter. You can view the codes that would be transferred in Figure 8-34.

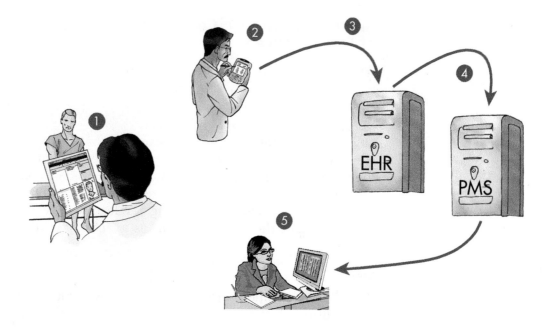

► Figure 8-35 **Flow of procedures posted from EHR to billing.**

Figure 8-35 illustrates the typical method of posting charges from an EHR to a Practice Management billing module. The steps include the following:

1. Clinician documents encounter at point of care.

2. EHR calculates E&M code.

3. Clinician clicks button labeled "Post To Encounter."

4. EHR adds procedure codes to encounter note and transfers CPT-4 and ICD-9-CM codes to the practice management system.

5. A billing or coding specialist reviews the "pending" charges, adds modifiers or other information, and posts them.

Figure 8-36 shows a practice management billing screen used to post charges transferred from the EHR after being reviewed by a billing or coding specialist.

► Figure 8-36 **Practice management system posting E&M code from EHR.**

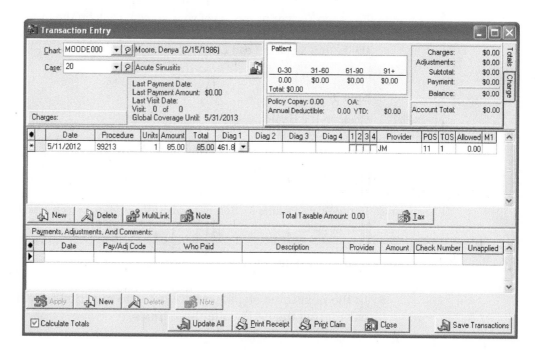

Guided Exercise 41: Counseling More Than 50% of Face-to-Face Time

When counseling or coordination of care represents more than 50% of the face-to-face time of the visit, time becomes a key or controlling factor to the level of E&M services.

You will recall from the previous exercise that the patient has been smoking since she was twenty. The clinician spent about 10 minutes of time counseling the patient on the need to stop using tobacco and discussing possible strategies she might use to quit. This extra time spent counseling causes the visit to take longer. In this exercise you are going to reload the encounter, reenter the history, and recalculate the code using time as a factor.

Step 1

If the Student Edition software is not currently running on your system, start it at this time.

Perform the following tasks even if the patient encounter used in the previous exercise is still displayed on your screen. This will refresh the encounter and eliminate the changes you made in the previous exercise.

From the Select Menu, click Patient, and from the Patient Selector window select "Denya Moore."

From the Select Menu, click Existing Encounter, and from the Encounter Selector window select "5/11/2012 10:45 AM (Office Visit)." If you have difficulty, refer to Figure 8-3 at the beginning of this chapter.

Do not run the E&M Calculator yet.

Step 2

From the Toolbar at the top of your screen, click on the button labeled "List." When the Lists Manager window shown in Figure 8-22 is displayed, select "Adult URI" and click the button labeled "Load List."

Step 3

Click on the Hx tab.

Locate and click on the following History finding:

  ● (red button) current smoker

In the Entry Details section at the bottom of your screen type **6 years** in the field labeled "Duration."

If you have difficulty, refer to Figure 8-25 in the previous exercise.

In the next three steps, you are going to experiment with the Time function, calculating the E&M code three times.

Step 4

Locate and click on the E&M button in the Toolbar at the top of your screen to invoke the Evaluation and Management Calculator window. The Problem Screening checklist window is displayed.

Locate and click the boxes for the following:

✓ Active

✓ New Problem

When the Evaluation and Management Calculator is displayed, locate and click the button labeled "Calculate E&M Code."

Note that the Calculated E&M Code is 99212, the same as it was in the beginning of the previous exercises.

Step 5

Locate the check box used to indicate that counseling (or coordination of care) exceeded 50% of the face-to-face time for the visit. The box is circled in red in Figure 8-37. Click your mouse on the field and a check mark will appear.

Click your mouse on the down arrow button in the field labeled "Total face to face or Floor time," and select "10 minutes" from the drop-down list.

Click the button labeled "Calculate E&M Code." The code should still calculate as 99212. Notice that the code did **not** change, even though the box labeled ">50%" was checked.

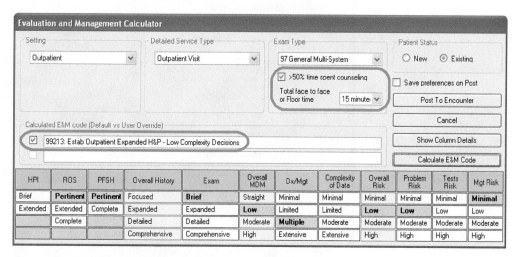

▶ Figure 8-37 **E&M code recalculated using time as a factor.**

Step 6

Click your mouse on the down arrow button in the field labeled "Total face to face or Floor time," and this time select 15 minutes from the drop-down list.

Click the button labeled "Calculate E&M Code."

Compare your screen to Figure 8-37. The newly calculated code on your screen should be 99213.

In step 5, the code did not increase to a higher level because the E&M Calculator has a minimum amount of time expected to complete each level of exam. Refer back to the table in Figure 8-21. In the right column, the standard amount of time is shown for each code. The E&M code 99212 has a minimum face-to-face time of 10 minutes, whereas the next higher level E&M code, 99213, has a minimum face-to-face time of 15 minutes.

When the face-to-face time for this exam was set at less than 15 minutes, the E&M Calculator did not increase the code to the next level. Once you increased the amount of time, and checked the box labeled ">50% time spent counseling," time became the controlling or key component.

Locate and click on the button labeled "Post To Encounter."

Step 7

The E&M description, code, time, and justification are posted to your encounter, as shown in Figure 8-38. Remember you can only use time to increase the level of E&M code when the clinician has spent more that 50% of the face-to-face time in counseling or coordination of care. In Denya's case, the clinician spent >10 minutes of the total 15 minutes in counseling.

▶ Figure 8-38 **Encounter note showing counseling time >50%.**

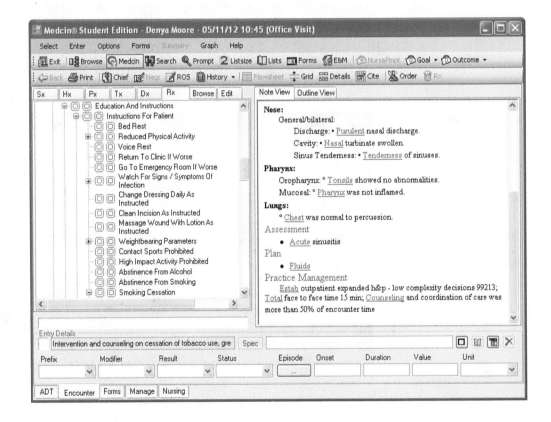

Remember that the guideline also states: ". . . the record should describe the counseling and/or activities to coordinate care."[5] This means that whenever you use this feature in a medical office, you must add a finding or free text to describe the counseling.

---

[5]Ibid.

Step 8

To clear the Adult URI list, click on the button labeled "Medcin," which is highlighted on the Toolbar in Figure 8-38.

Click on the Rx tab.

Locate "Basic Management Procedures and Services" and click on the small plus sign.

Scroll the screen to locate and expand the tree for "Education and Instructions" and then for "Instructions to the Patient."

Scroll the screen to locate and expand the tree for "Smoking cessation" and then for "with intervention and counseling."

Locate and click on the following finding:

● (red button) Greater than 10 minutes

Compare your screen to Figure 8-39.

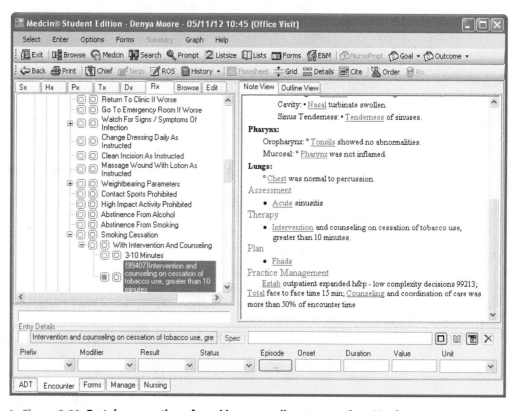

▶ Figure 8-39 Rx tab—cessation of smoking counseling greater than 10 minutes.

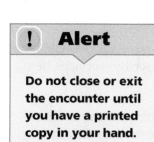
Step 9

Click on the Print button on the Toolbar at the top of your screen to invoke the Print Data window.

Be certain there is a check mark in the box next to "Current Encounter" and then click on the appropriate button to either print or export a file, as directed by your instructor.

Compare your printout or file output to Figure 8-40. If it is correct, hand it in to your instructor. If there are any differences, review the previous steps in the exercise and find your error.

Student: *your name or ID here*
Patient: Denya Moore: F: 2/15/1986: 5/11/2012 10:45 AM
Chief complaint
The Chief Complaint is: Patient reports stuffy sinus.
Personal history
Behavioral: Current smoker for 6 years.
Review of systems
Head: Sinus pain.
Physical findings
Ears:
　　General/bilateral:
　　　　Tympanic Membrane: ° Both tympanic membranes were normal.
Nose:
　　General/bilateral:
　　　　Discharge: • Purulent nasal discharge.
　　　　Cavity: • Nasal turbinate swollen.
　　　　Sinus Tenderness: • Tenderness of sinuses.
Pharynx:
　　Oropharynx: ° Tonsils showed no abnormalities.
　　Mucosal: ° Pharynx was not inflamed.
Lungs:
　　° Chest was normal to percussion.
Assessment
　　• Acute sinusitis
Therapy
　　• Intervention and counseling on cessation of tobacco use, greater than 10 minutes.
Plan
　　• Fluids
Practice Management
　　Estab outpatient expanded h&p - low complexity decisions 99213; Total face to face time 15 min;
　　Counseling and coordination of care was more than 50% of encounter time.

▶ Figure 8-40 **Printed encounter note for Denya Moore with counseling finding and time added.**

Chapter Eight Summary

CPT-4 and ICD-9-CM codes are national standards that are required on insurance claims for outpatient and other services.

For both inpatient and outpatient facilities, the use of the correct ICD-9-CM code on a claim serves to explain or justify the medical reason for the services being billed.

Reimbursement for most inpatient hospitals is based entirely on the diagnosis-related group (DRG) determined from the primary and secondary diagnoses assigned by the attending physician.

Outpatient billing requires one or more ICD-9-CM codes to be assigned to every procedure and the diagnosis must be appropriate for the procedure.

The use of HCPCS and CPT-4 codes for procedures is also required. CPT stands for Current Procedural Terminology. It was developed and is maintained by the AMA.

A group of the CPT-4 codes called Evaluation and Management (E&M) codes is used to bill for nearly every kind of patient encounter.

There are separate categories of E&M codes for different locations such as outpatient, inpatient hospital exams, nursing home visits, consults, emergency room doctors, and so on.

There are four levels of E&M codes within each category. The levels represent the least complicated exam (level 1) to the most complex exam (level 4), with higher levels paying the provider more.

The medical record for the encounter must support the level of E&M code billed with documented findings. An EHR can accurately calculate the correct level of E&M code from the findings that are documented.

Seven components are used in defining the level of E&M services:

- History
- Examination
- Medical decision making
- Counseling
- Coordination of care
- Nature of presenting problem
- Time.

The first three of these components are called key components. Each of the key components has subcomponents, called elements, that determine the level of the component. Once the level of each of the key components is determined, the results are evaluated to calculate the correct level of E&M code.

Time is used to adjust the level of the E&M code only when counseling/coordination of care exceeds 50% of the face-to-face time.

Because the level of E&M code is dependent on the levels of multiple key components, merely adding more findings to only one key component may bring that component to a higher level, but that does not necessarily mean that the visit as a whole will qualify for the higher level E&M code.

Testing Your Knowledge of Chapter 8

1. What does the acronym E&M stand for?
2. How many levels are there for a category of E&M code?
3. Name the three key components of an E&M code.
4. How many levels are there for each key component?
5. How many key components determine the level of E&M code for an established patient?

Write the definitions for the following History acronyms:

6. HPI _____
7. ROS _____
8. PFSH _____
9. Explain how the level of a general multisystem examination is determined.
10. What determines the level of risk?
11. What makes up face-to-face time?
12. When does time become a factor in determining the level of E&M code?
13. What does the E&M button on the Toolbar do?
14. How do you record an E&M code in a patient encounter note?
15. You should have produced two narrative documents of patient encounters. If you have not already done so, hand these in to your instructor with this test. The printed encounter notes will count as a portion of your grade.

Chapter Nine

Comprehensive Evaluation

This comprehensive evaluation will enable you and your instructor to determine your understanding of the material in this course that was presented in Chapters 1 through 8. Complete both the written test and the hands-on exercise provided below. Depending on the time provided, it may be necessary to do this in two separate sessions. Your instructor will advise you. Do not begin the critical thinking exercise if there will not be enough class time to complete it.

Part 1: Written Exam

You may run the Student Edition software and use your mouse on the screen to answer the following questions:

Give a brief description of the purpose of each of the following coding systems:

1. Medcin

2. CPT-4

3. ICD-9-CM

4. Explain the difference between an EHR nomenclature and a billing code set.

5. Describe how to retrieve a previous patient encounter.

6. Which screen do you use to set the reason for the visit?

7. How do you load a list?

8. How do you enter vital signs?

Write the meaning of each of the following medical abbreviations:

9. ROS _____

10. Hx _____

11. HEENT _____

12. Dx _____

13. PFSH _____

14. URI _____

15. E&M _____

16. Describe how to record a test that was performed.

17. How many levels are there for a category of E&M codes?

18. Name the key components of an E&M code.

19. What Entry Details field is used with a finding to indicate a "possible" diagnosis?

20. What determines the E&M level of risk?

21. Where are "bullets" as used in E&M calculations?

Describe the purpose of the following buttons on the Medcin Toolbar:

22. Prompt _____

23. Order _____

24. Listsize _____

25. Rx _____

26. Search _____

27. Negs _____

28. ROS _____

29. E&M _____

30. Explain the difference between calculating the E&M level of a general multisystem examination and a single-organ examination.

Part 2: Critical Thinking Exercise

The following exercise will use features of the software with which you have become familiar. Complete each step in sequential order using the instructions and other information provided.

When you have finished the complete exercise, print out the encounter note and hand it to your instructor. Do not begin the hands-on exercise if there will not be enough class time to complete it.

Critical Thinking Exercise 42: Examination of a Patient with Asthma

George Blackstone is a 30-year-old established patient with possible mild asthma who comes to the office complaining of awakening in the night short of breath. George does not smoke, but he is exposed to second-hand smoke and has pets in the house.

In this exercise, you use the skills you have acquired to document this exam.

Step 1

If you have not already done so, start the Student Edition software.

Click Select on the Menu bar, and then click Patient.

In the Patient Selection window, locate and click on "George Blackstone."

Step 2

Click Select on the Menu bar, and then click New Encounter.

Select the date "May 14, 2012," the time "9:15 AM," and the reason "10 Minute Visit."

Make certain that you set the date and reason correctly. Compare your screen to the date, time, and reason given above before clicking on the OK button.

Step 3

Enter the chief complaint by locating the button in the Toolbar labeled "Chief" and clicking on it.

In the dialog window that will open, type **Patient reports waking at night short of breath**.

When you have finished typing, click on the button labeled "Close the note form."

Step 4

Begin the visit by taking George's vital signs and medical history.

Use the form labeled "Vitals," which you will select from the Forms Manager.

Enter George's vital signs in the corresponding fields on the form as follows:

Temperature:	**98.6**
Respiration:	**28**
Pulse:	**78**
BP:	**120/80**
Height:	**71**
Weight:	**175**

When you have finished, check your work. If it is correct, proceed to step 5.

Step 5

Remain on the Forms tab. Take the patient's medical history by using the Short Intake form.

Locate and click on the button labeled "Forms" in the Toolbar at the top of your screen to invoke the Forms Manager window again.

Locate and click on the form labeled "Short Intake" as you have done in previous exercises.

Step 6

When the Short Intake form is displayed, locate and click on the tab labeled "Medical History."

Enter the Dx History and Family History by clicking on the Y (yes) check box or the N (no) check box for the following items:

Diagnosis	Dx Hist	Family Hist
Angina	✓ N	✓ N
Asthma	✓ Y	✓ N
Bronchitis	✓ Y	✓ N
Cancer	✓ N	✓ N
Congestive Heart Failure	✓ N	✓ N
Coronary Artery Disease	✓ N	✓ N
Diabetes	✓ N	✓ N
Heart Attack	✓ N	✓ N
Hypertension	✓ N	✓ N
Migraine Headache	✓ N	✓ N
Peptic Ulcer	✓ N	✓ N
Reflux	✓ N	✓ N
Stroke	✓ N	✓ N

Complete the rest of his Medical History on the right side of the form by locating and clicking on the check boxes as follows:

Currently Taking Medication?	✓ N
Recent Exposure–Contagious	✓ N
Recent History of Travel?	✓ N
Recent Medical Examination	✓ Y
Recent X-Ray	✓ N
Recent ECG?	✓ N
Allergies	✓ Y
Allergy To Drugs	✓ N
Tobacco Use	✓ N
Alcohol Use	✓ Y

When you have finished, check your work. If it is correct, click on the Encounter tab at the bottom of the screen.

Step 7

Locate and click on the Lists button in the Toolbar at the top of your screen. The Lists Manager window will be invoked.

Two fields at the top of the Lists Manager window organize the display of List names, filtering them by Owner and Group. The Student Edition has two groups, "All" and "Student Edition."

Click on the down arrow in the Group field and select the Group "Student Edition." Locate and highlight the list named "Asthma." Click your mouse on the button labeled "Load List."

Step 8

The left pane should be on the Sx tab. If it is not, click on the tab labeled "Sx."

Locate and click on the following symptom findings:

- (red button) awaking at night short of breath

The text will change to Paroxysmal Nocturnal Dyspnea.

Step 9

Locate and click on the ROS button in the Toolbar at the top of your screen.

Verify that the ROS button is depressed.

Locate and click on the button labeled "Negs" in the Toolbar at the top of your screen.

All unselected symptoms findings will be set by the Auto Negative feature.

Step 10

Next, click on the Hx tab to enter the patient's history. Note that "No family history of Asthma" was already set via the Short Intake form.

Locate and click on the following findings:

- (blue button) Previous Hospitalization for pulmonary problem
- (red button) Exposure to Second-hand Cigarette Smoke
- (red button) Exposure to Dust Mites
- (red button) Exposure to Animal Dander

Step 11

Click on the Px tab to document the physical exam. Notice that the findings from the Vitals form are already displayed.

Locate and highlight the finding: "Intranasal polyp mm."

In the Entry Details section of your screen, locate the field labeled "Value," and enter the numeric value **0.2** (two-tenths). Then press the Enter key.

Click the drop-down button in the Units field and change the unit from mm to **cm**.

The finding text should change to read ".2 cm intranasal polyp."

Step 12

Locate the button labeled "Negs" in the Toolbar and click it once.

Px findings not previously set will be set by the Auto Negative feature.

Step 13

Click on Tx tab.

Locate and highlight "CBC with Differential," and click on the order button on the Toolbar.

Expand the tree of findings for Pulmonary Function Tests.

Locate and highlight "Spirometry" and click on the order button.

Verify that both tests appear in the plan before proceeding.

Step 14

Click on the Dx tab.

Click on the plus sign for history of Asthma.

Locate and click on the following finding:

- (red button) Intermittent

Click the down arrow button in the prefix field. Select the prefix "possible" from the drop-down list displayed.

Step 15

Click on the Rx tab.

Expand the tree for Environmental Control Measures.

Locate and click on the following findings:

- (red button) Frequent vacuuming
- (red button) Avoid Allergens
- (red button) Patient Education – Asthma
- (red button) Follow-up visit

Step 16

Enter a prescription.

Expand the tree for Bronchodilators.

Locate and highlight "Albuterol."

Click on the Rx button in the Toolbar. The prescription writer window will be invoked.

Step 17

In the Rx Dosage Inquiry window, locate and click on the following Sig:

"90 microgram puffs 1 inh prn DSP1."

When the Rx Brand Inquiry window is displayed, position your mouse over the brand "Proventil" and click your mouse button.

Locate the field labeled "Generic Allowed."

Click your mouse in the white circle next to "Yes." It should then be filled in.

Review the completed prescription. If anything is incorrect, click on the button labeled "Rx Inquiry" to correct it.

Locate and click on the button labeled "Save Rx."

Step 18

Locate and click on the button labeled "E&M" in the Toolbar at the top of your screen.

The Problem Screening checklist should be invoked.

Locate and check the box:

✓ Chronic

Click the OK button. The E&M Calculator window should be invoked.

Step 19

! Alert

Do not close or exit the encounter until you have a printed copy in your hand. *You will lose your work if you exit before printing.*

Locate the Patient Status section in the upper right corner of the E&M Calculator window. Click your mouse in the white circle labeled "Existing." It should then be filled in.

Locate and click your mouse on the down arrow button in the field labeled "Total face to face or Floor time." Select "10 minutes" from the drop-down list.

Locate and click on the button labeled "Calculate E&M Code." The calculated E&M code field should display "99213: Estab Outpatient Expanded H&P—Low Complexity Decisions."

If this is the code displayed in your window, locate and click on the button labeled "Post To Encounter." If this is not the code calculated, click on the Cancel button, and review the previous steps to find your error.

Step 20

Click on the Print button on the Toolbar at the top of your screen to invoke the Print Data window.

Be certain there is a check mark in the box next to "Current Encounter" and then click on the appropriate button to either print or export a file, as directed by your instructor.

Compare your printout or file output to Figure 9-1. If it is correct, hand it in to your instructor. If there are any differences, review the previous steps in the exercise and find your error.

Student: *your name or ID here*
Patient: George Blackstone: M: 10/10/1981: 5/14/2012 09:15 AM

Chief complaint

The Chief Complaint is: Patient reports waking at night short of breath.

History of present illness

George Blackstone is a 28 year old male.
He reported: Paroxysmal nocturnal dyspnea.

Past medical/surgical history

Reported History:
Medical: No previous hospitalization for a pulmonary problem. A recent medical examination.
Medications: Not taking medication.
Tests: No chest x-ray was performed and an ECG was not performed.
Exposure: No exposure to a contagious disease.
Environmental Exposure: Secondhand cigarette smoke exposure, exposure to dust mites, and animal dander.

Diagnosis History:
No coronary artery disease
No angina pectoris
No acute myocardial infarction
No congestive heart failure.
No hypertension.
Bronchitis
Asthma.
No esophageal reflux
No peptic ulcer.
No diabetes mellitus.
No migraine headache
No stroke syndrome.
No cancer

Personal history

Behavioral: No tobacco use.
Alcohol: Alcohol use.
Travel: No travel.

Family history

No coronary artery disease
No angina pectoris
No acute myocardial infarction
No congestive heart failure
No hypertension
No bronchitis
No asthma
No esophageal reflux
No peptic ulcer
No diabetes mellitus
No migraine headache
No stroke syndrome
No cancer.

Review of systems

Systemic: Not feeling tired or poorly. No fever and no recent weight loss.
Head: No headache and no sinus pain.

Continued on the following page...

▶ Figure 9-1a **Printed encounter note for George Blackstone (page 1 of 2).**

Eyes: No watery discharge from eyes. No red eyes.
Otolaryngeal: No nasal passage blockage and no sore throat.
Cardiovascular: No chest pain or discomfort.
Pulmonary: Not feeling congested in the chest, no dyspnea, no cough, no hemoptysis, and no wheezing.

Physical findings

Vital Signs:

Vital Signs/Measurements	Value	Normal Range
Oral temperature	98.6 F	97.6 - 99.6
RR	28 breaths/min	18 - 26
PR	78 bpm	50 - 100
Blood pressure	120/80 mmHg	100-120/60-80
Weight	175 lbs	125 - 225
Height	71 in	65.35 - 74.02

° No pulsus paradoxus was noted.

Eyes:
> General/bilateral:
>> External: ° No petechiae in the conjunctiva.

Nose:
> General/bilateral:
>> Discharge: ° No rhinorrhea.
>> Cavity: • 0.2 cm intranasal polyp.

Lymph Nodes:
> ° Normal.

Lungs:
> ° Respiration rhythm and depth was normal. ° Respiratory movements were normal.
> ° Chest was normal to percussion. ° No decrease in breath sounds was heard.
> ° No wheezing was heard. ° No rhonchi were heard. ° No prolonged expiratory time.
> ° No rales/crackles were heard.

Cardiovascular:
> Murmurs: ° No murmurs were heard.

Abdomen:
> Palpation: ° No abdominal tenderness.

Skin:
> ° No cyanosis.

Assessment
> • Possible intermittent asthma

Therapy
> • Frequent vacuuming.
> • Avoid exposure to allergens.
> • Follow-up visit.

Allergies
> An allergy. No known drug allergies.

Counseling/Education
> • Patient education about asthma

Plan
> • CBC with differential
> • Spirometry
> • Albuterol
> 90 ug puffs (1 inh prn) DISP:1 inhal Refill:3 Generic:Y Using:Proventil Mfg: Schering

Practice Management
> Estab outpatient expanded h&p - low complexity decisions 99213; Total face to face time ten min

▶ **Figure 9-1b Printed encounter note for George Blackstone (page 2 of 2).**

Index